HEALTH ECONOMICS: Prospects for the Future

The purpose of this book is to review the current state of health economics and look forward to developments over the next 25 years. The coverage is international, individual countries, areas and the World Health Organization, being considered by world experts. Other topics examined include cost-benefit analysis and issues concerning the pharmaceutical industry. The book should represent a major statement of the field, of interest to economists and health planners.

Edited by George Teeling Smith, Director,
Office of Health Economics, London

HEALTH ECONOMICS:
Prospects for the Future

Edited by GEORGE TEELING SMITH

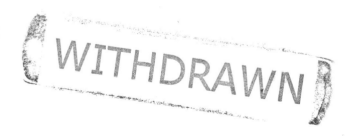

CROOM HELM
London ● New York ● Sydney

© 1987 Office of Health Economics

Croom Helm Ltd, Provident House, Burrell Row,
Beckenham, Kent BR3 1AT

Croom Helm Australia, 44–50 Waterloo Road,
North Ryde, 2113, New South Wales

Published in the USA by Croom Helm
in association with Methuen, Inc.
29 West 35th Street
New York, NY10001

British Library Cataloguing in Publication Data

Health economics: prospects for the future.
    1. Medical economics
    I. Teeling-Smith, George
    338.4′73621   RA410

    ISBN 0-7099-1958-1

Library of Congress Cataloging-in-Publication Data

Health economics.

    Includes index.
    1. Medical economics. I. Smith, George Teeling,
1928– . [DNLM: 1. Economics, Medical — trends.
W 74 H4355]
RA410.H415 1987   338.4′73621   87-8998
ISBN 0-7099-1958-1

Filmset by Mayhew Typesetting, Bristol, England
Printed and bound in Great Britain
by Billings & Sons Limited, Worcester.

Contents

Preface

When reading through the various chapters on this book, one simple message is clear. Health economics is a growth industry. As the gap between what is technologically possible in health care and what is practically affordable widens, it will become more and more important to ensure that the most economic use is made of scarce health care resources. But there may also be a second reason why health economics is going to become more important. This is simply because it seems inevitable that health care is going to absorb a greater proportion of national wealth in the future. The present fashion is for 'cost containment', and some people predict that health care expenditure has reached its ceiling. However those of us with longer experience in the field can remember exactly the same crisis about 'excessive expenditure' on health in the 1950s. At that time, too, people believed that health care expenditure was out of control. Since then, however, health has doubled its share of national income in most advanced countries. It seems very probable that similar growth is going to continue in the future.

The driving forces behind this higher expenditure are threefold. First, there are the undoubted advances which will continue to take place in medical technology. A few of these will save health care expenditure, but the majority will add to demands for resources. Second, there is the changing demographic pattern (itself a result of this technological progress) which is greatly increasing the numbers of very frail elderly people in all our populations. Third, there is the question of public expectations. Increasingly people are going to want a better quality of life in health terms, if necessary at the expense of material well-being.

The late Lord Vaizey put his finger on the key issue in this context. He could not understand why the 'health care explosion' was seen as a 'problem', when a similarly explosive growth in expenditure on home electronics, for example, was greeted as an economic triumph. The answer, of course, is that health care costs are shared, whereas other forms of material consumption are paid for individually. A person buys his own television set, but expects other taxpayers or insured people to share the cost of his hospital treatment.

However it seems unlikely that this economic situation will in fact result in a containment of health care costs in the future. I have recently predicted that the United States, at least, may be spending 20 per cent of gross domestic product on health care by the early 2000s. If this seems improbable in 1987, it must be remembered that few people would have predicted in the 1960s that the United States would already be spending about 11 per cent of GDP on health by the 1980s.

If this prediction is realistic it helps to underline the future importance of health economics. The alternatives to a growth in expenditure would be restriction on technological progress of even compulsory euthansia. It is unlikely, in reality, that the electorate in any country would vote for either of these choices. Instead, they are likely to accept that the best use should be made of increasing health expenditures — and that means a growing reliance on health economics, which is the recurring theme of this book.

George Teeling Smith

Contributors

Professor Brian Abel-Smith, Professor of Social Administration, London School of Economics, and Political Science, UK

Martin Buxton, Director, Health Economics Research Group, Brunel University, UK

Professor Michael Cooper, Professor of Economics, University of Otago, New Zealand

Professor A.J. Culyer, Professor of Economics, University of York, UK

Dr Thi Dao, Health Policy Analyst, Syntex Corporation, USA

Dr Michael Drummond, Acting Director, Health Services Management Centre, University of Birmingham, UK

Professor Alain Enthoven, Professor of Public and Private Management, Stanford University, USA

Professor Shiro Fujino, Professor of Economics, Chuo University, Japan

Professor Ronald Hansen, Merrell Dow Associate Professor of Pharmacy Administration, Ohio State University, USA

Professor Bengt Jönsson, Professor of Economics, Linköping University, Sweden

Professor Alan Maynard, Professor of Economics and Director, Centre for Health Economics, University of York, UK

Professor Frank Münnich, Director, Medizinsch Pharmazeutische Studiengesellschaft, Mainz, FRG

Dr Simone Sandier, Health Economist, CREDES Paris, France

Professor George Teeling Smith, Director, Office of Health Economics, London, UK

Dr Klaus von Grebmer, Health Economist, CIBA Geigy, Basel, Switzerland

Nicholas Wells, Associate Director, Office of Health Economics, London, UK

Dr Gail Wilensky, Vice President, Division of Health Affairs, Project HOPE, USA

Professor Alan Williams, Professor of Economics, University of York, UK

Dr Herbert Zöllner, Regional Office for Health Economics, WHO European Office, Copenhagen, Denmark

1

Prospects for the Future: an Introductory Overview

George Teeling Smith

THE BACKGROUND

Twenty-five years ago, in 1962, health economics was in its infancy. Indeed, only a few years earlier the British economist Dennis Lees had been told by his colleagues that he should not study health at all. 'It was not a subject for economic analysis.' However he and several other pioneering economists persisted and the discipline of health economics was duly born.

In the early days, in Britain at least, the economic debate was mainly political. Statistics were gathered on the one hand to show the advantages of 'socialised medicine' and on the other to defend the private market for medical care. By the time that the Office of Health Economics was set up in 1962, however, it was becoming clear that this political argument was largely sterile. It started to become clear that the economic problems surrounding health services transcended political frontiers. Shortages and inefficiencies were endemic regardless of the political system.

Nevertheless in the early 1960s health economics still consisted largely of marshalling statistics about expenditures on health care and of the measurement of medical activities. Numbers of doctors, nurses and other staff, and their types of activity, were systematically monitored. On expenditure, it was pointed out that Britain, so far from having had a profligate National Health Service, had actually been reducing the percentage of gross national product devoted to health care during the 1950s. As far as patients were concerned, in a monumental econometric analysis, Martin Feldstein, on a visit from the United States, showed that National Health Service districts which had larger numbers of hospital beds admitted more patients and tended to keep them in hospital for longer

1

Figure 1.1: The 'black box' of health economics

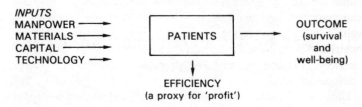

(Feldstein, 1967). It was clear that Parkinson's Law was operating. However during this phase in the development of health economics little attention was paid to the outcome of therapies, except, notably, in terms of global analysis of falling mortality rates due to the 'therapeutic revolution' since the Second World War.

The present approach to the discipline started to emerge in the 1970s, when much more objective and critical debate began to take place about the relationship between heatlh service costs and activities on the one hand and health care outcomes on the other. At the Office of Health Economics, the subject was looked at as the sort of magic black box shown in Figure 1.1. Outcomes were related to inputs in a systematic way, and their relationship provided some measure of the efficiency of the health service.

On the political front, it became clear that a conventional market was impossible for health care, for two very simple reasons. First, those most in need were those least able to pay. And second, the costs of treatment could often be prohibitive even for the relatively affluent. Chronic treatment or care which might cost tens of thousands of dollars or pounds each year would soon be financially crippling even for rich middle class families. Nevertheless, it was equally clear that a monolithic bureaucracy, such as Britain's National Health Service, lacked some of the necessary economic incentives to ensure the most efficient use of limited resources.

During the 1970s this led to a debate about the possible advantages of the type of health insurance schemes operated in Europe, as opposed to the tax-funded and centrally controlled system in Britain. However, like the earlier private market versus socialised medicine debate this too proved a sterile basis for discussion. It soon became clear that the method of funding health services — insurance as against taxation — was of little importance. The Europeans raised more money through their insurance schemes, and hence some visible signs of shortage (such as hospital waiting lists) were absent.

But overall, the economic problems of balancing limited resources against virtually unlimited demands existed throughout all the European countries, and not just in Britain. The higher spending on health care as a proportion of national wealth in other European countries was in the main an indication of their greater affluence. The richer a nation becomes, the higher *percentage* of this wealth it devotes to health.

Thus by the 1980s, the health economics debate had become a very great deal more sophisticated than it had been twenty years earlier. It had also become less overtly political. The sharp differences between the left and the right, which had seemed to be central to health economics issues in the 1960s have by now become peripheral. No political party holds the solution to the central dilemma, which is that no country could ever afford to do everything that is technologically possible in medicine.

It is against this background that the present book reviews the future of health economics over the next 25 years, and looks from various points of view at the issues which now seem relevant to the organisation of health services. On the following pages, by way of introduction, there is brief reference to seven of these issues, which seem likely to be the subject of continuing study over the next quarter of a century.

PATTERNS OF EXPENDITURE

It has already been pointed out that richer nations tend to spend a higher percentage of their national wealth on health. Table 1.1 shows the percentage of Gross Domestic Product devoted to health in eleven comparable developed countries in 1982. A question for the future is whether the poorer countries such as Britain can catch up again with richer countries such as Sweden and the United States.

However a very much greater question mark hangs over the relative expenditures in the developed and the developing world. Although countries such as Britain are experiencing severe shortages of medical care, compared for example with the United States, the real problem of shortage arises most acutely in the Third World. Predominantly, it is matter of overall poverty. There is a dramatic contrast in expenditure on health between the richer and poorer countries of the world. Even the simple crude figures for life expectancy shown in Table 1.2 indicate very clearly the resulting difference in health status.

Table 1.1: Health as a percentage of GDP, 1982

USA	10.6
Sweden	9.3
France	9.3
Netherlands	8.7
Germany	8.2
Switzerland	7.8
Italy	7.2
Denmark	6.8
Japan	6.6
Belgium	6.2
UK	5.9

Source: OECD.

Table 1.2: Life expectancy at birth, 1977

	Years
Japan	76
UK	73
France	73
Germany	72
Kuwait	69
Libya	55
Egypt	54
Saudi Arabia	48
Bangladesh	47
Ethiopia	39

Source: World Bank.

The World Health Organization is committed to the principle of 'Health for All by the Year 2000'. Table 1.2 indicates how difficult it will be to get anywhere near this praiseworthy objective within that given time scale. Health economists can do little to help except to point to the magnitude of the international political task. They can, however, draw attention to the biased allocation of the very limited health care resources in the Third World, where much is often spent on very advanced medical care in the urban setting and very little is devoted to the much greater medical needs in the poor rural areas.

This, again, however is a social and political issue as well as an economic one. A country such as India has about 50 million affluent citizens who expect a standard of medical care similar to that provided for the citizens of Europe or the United States. The fact that there are also about 700 million people living in abject poverty does not immediately reduce the expectations of the rich for Western standards of treatment. Nor is there much economic evidence that depriving the rich of their expected standard of care would automatically result in the poor receiving correspondingly better medical attention. Nevertheless, although health economists can do little to relieve the overall problems of poverty in the Third World, they could possibly develop new theories to help in the redistribution of resources between the most affluent and the least affluent sections of the world population. This is undoubtedly a challenge for the next 25 years. Certainly inequalities in medical care should continue to be a major preoccupation of health economists.

SYSTEMS OF PROVIDING MEDICAL CARE

It was pointed out in the brief introductory review that differences between systems of providing health care do not seem to play a central role in determining the quality of care. By and large, tax funded schemes, national health insurance schemes, social insurance or even private insurance all have their advantages and disadvantages. However, this does not mean that health economics has no place in the analysis of the relative effectiveness of different systems in a more detailed way. In the past, for example, Maynard and Ludbrook (1981) have usefully compared some different European systems. Their findings at least suggested, although they could not prove, that an element of private insurance in the Dutch system did not seem to disadvantage the poorer sectors of the community. More recently Ware and others (1986) in the United States have shown that payment of a fee for each item of service seems to ensure better care for the indigent sick than the alternative — a flat-rate prepaid health care scheme.

This debate in the United States between fee-for-item-of-service and the alternative Health Maintenance Organisation (HMO) approach to medical care is certain to be a burning issue for health economists in the years ahead. The HMO is in theory much better placed to concentrate on preventive medicine and to avoid 'unnecessary' treatments which a fee paid for each item may encourage. However Ware's findings seriously challenge the validity of the traditional conclusion that the HMO therefore provides more rational care. It looks as if, in practice, simply 'throwing money at a problem' may be the way to achieve the best care for those most in need. In the same study, treatment for the fee-for-service patients cost on average 40 per cent more than that for the HMO patients. Ironically, however, the rich and relatively healthy did not seem to benefit correspondingly from their extra services. It was only for the sick poor that a difference showed up.

Clearly this recent study from the United States underlines the role which analysis by health economists must play in the future in trying to identify the most efficient and most economical pattern for the provision of health care. No system is perfect at present, and further studies are urgently needed to help national governments or health care agencies to move towards more effective systems of providing health care.

THE ADVANTAGES OF AN 'INTERNAL MARKET'

Economists and politicians have regularly pointed out that there are in principle only two ways of allocating scarce resources. One is through the market place, where each individual can buy what he most wants with the finances which he has at his disposal. The other is through a central bureaucracy, in which individuals' private resources are collected by the government (for example, through taxes) and are spent centrally on the goods and services which the bureaucracy deems to be most valuable for the community as a whole. The latter system is often advocated on the grounds of greater 'fairness'. The services go to those in need rather than to those who have earned (or inherited) the resources to buy them. Nevertheless, fairness apart, the Western democracies have increasingly recognised that the bureaucratic method has two overwhelming disadvantages. First, it removes the personal economic incentive to create more wealth. Second, it has great scope for inefficiency. Without the measure of 'profit' (in whatever form) as an indicator of efficiency, it is extremely hard to identify (let alone reward) efficient performance or to eradicate inefficiency. Thus the objective of Western governments has been to create a basically fair society without the inbuilt efficiencies of a central bureaucracy.

Fairness is, of course, relative. No social system can make a plain girl beautiful or a stupid man clever. But it can try to minimise the relative advantages and disadvantages of different individuals, without at the same time removing individual incentives for maximum human achievement. Nowhere is the dilemma inherent in attempting to balance efficiency with fairness more dominant than

6

in health economics. The best solution which economists have had to offer so far is the concept of an 'internal market' in a fundamentally bureaucratic system for providing prepaid medical treatment and care. The idea is to introduce the incentive to efficiency which exists in the market place into a system of medical care which does not depend on an individual patient's ability to pay.

There are many different forms under discussion as to how this concept might be realised. One, which has been surrounded in controversy, is the 'voucher system' applied to both health and education. This gives each individual vouchers to cover the cost of their services, as far as possible in proportion to their need. With these vouchers they can shop around — in the same way that they could with ordinary money — to 'buy' the most attractive education or medical treatment which they can find. There are many difficulties with the system, but economists should not abandon the principle simply because it has problems. The role of the health economist should be to solve problems, not merely to identify them.

Another approach to the market system, under a prepaid health care plan, is the Health Maintenance Organisation found in the United States. Again this is a concept — despite its limitations — which deserves further analysis and modification. Yet a further alternative, which has been suggested by Maynard and discussed by the Office of Health Economics (Teeling Smith, 1984) is to put the 'purchasing power' for medical care into the hands of the general practitioners or family doctors. Using government funds, within certain predetermined limits, they would then 'buy' the best possible medical treatments for the patients under their care. Again this is an important area for economic experiment and analysis in the years ahead.

Overall, it is clear that health economists have a great deal to offer in attempting to match fairness with efficiency in health care, under a variety of different social and political systems. The whole field of competition versus regulation is a fruitful one for economic analysis.

MEASUREMENT OF HEALTH BENEFITS

Historically, up to the 1970s, the measurement of benefits of medical care was largely confined to analysis of life expectancy and patterns of mortality. Other measures of 'benefit', such as numbers of operations performed or numbers of patients admitted to hospital, were clearly in reality measures of activity and not of well-being. No patient would feel better off because he was operated on twice instead of once!

By the 1980s, therefore, a new approach to the measurement of benefits from medical treatment had been developed. This concentrated not only on survival but also, centrally, on the quality of life. Two broad approaches have been used. The first is based on a 'health profile', which measures the degree of the patient's well-being for such parameters as pain, energy, sleep and mobility. The other is based on a 'health index'. This defines a series of 'health states' and gives each of the states a score relative to the others. This whole approach is discussed fully in Professor Williams' chapter, so there is no need to elaborate it here.

There is no doubt that measurements of the quality of life are going to play a very important part in the development of health economics over the next 25 years. However, many questions remain to be answered.

Can, for example, longevity and the degree of well-being be successfully combined into the units of 'quality adjusted life years' (QALYs) which have so far been used? Are measurements of well-being using a health index analogous to units of weight, where two one pound units unambiguously equal one two pound unit? Or are they more analogous to units of temperature, where two days with a temperature of 15°C cannot in any sense be equated to one day of 30°C! These are important questions for health economists to answer in the years ahead.

The answers are urgently needed, because already economists are attempting to relate units of health care benefit to units of cost, to provide what can be called a 'cost-utility' analysis. It will perhaps be even more useful to be able to balance generally accepted units of well-being against measurements of the risk associated with treatment, to produce a 'risk-benefit' analysis. This is needed to put much publicised risks into perspective.

TOWARDS A FUNDAMENTAL THEORY

So far, these glimpses of the future have concerned quite concrete problems. Another role for health economists in the latter part of this century and the early part of the next would be to work towards a more fundamental economic theory of health care. To a large extent this concerns the distinction between the standard economic concept of 'demand' and the much more nebulous social concept of 'need'. Demand is determined by a person's individual desires and their ability to pay. These two factors vary in their importance according to the type of goods or service on offer. Thus in the Western world the demand for bread is determined predominantly by how much individuals choose to eat in relation to alternative basic foods, such as potatoes or biscuits. The relative price of bread, biscuits and potatoes is comparatively unimportant. On the other hand demand for *haute couture* clothes is determined predominantly by the number of people able and willing to pay for this particular form of luxury. Price starts to play a major part in determining demand.

In the same way, the nature of demand for health care can also be affected both by the desire to obtain it and by the ability to pay, if it is left in the private market place. However most societies have decided that the ability to pay should no longer be a criterion for a person's ability to obtain medical treatment. Hence the existence of prepaid schemes such as the British National Health Service or Medicare in the United States.

But once a service is available at zero price, standard economic theory breaks down. There is no price-regulator to determine demand. As indicated earlier, the availability of the treatment often becomes a bureaucratic decision rather than a market-place one. And in determining availability the bureaucrats start to take need instead of demand into account. Now the problem in economic terms is that need is much harder to define than demand. No one needs even bread, if potatoes and biscuits are available instead. Certainly no one 'needs' a *haute couture* dress, in an objective absolute sense, although a lady attending an important social reception may certainly feel that her need is absolute as far as she is concerned. Thus economists have to start to think in terms of relative need for health care, and to start to put values on degrees of need. At the same time, if human values and personal freedoms are to be taken into account, it is impossible wholly to neglect demand in relation to health care.

A very important transition in health economics is already starting to take place in this context. Whereas until the 1970s, the doctors were regarded as the arbiters of medical need, it is now being recognised that patients may know better for themselves what form of treatment they would actually like. It may not always be the type of treatment which would give the 'best' outcome in medical terms. This links back to measurement of the patients' quality of life. An appropriate objective for health economics in the future must depend

9

on maximising the *patients'* well-being, regardless of what doctors feel would be best for them. This supremacy of the customer — which is fundamental to much of economics — is sometimes difficult for an essentially authoritarian medical profession to accept. And of course in health economics the principle of the supremacy of the individual must also be integrated into a system which maximises the well-being of the community as a whole. All of this raises difficult philosophical problems which the health economists must face up to as their own profession develops in the years ahead.

THE INTEGRATION OF ECONOMICS AND MEDICINE

Another important objective for health economists is to work more closely with doctors in the future. Already in the measurement of quality of life, for example, some doctors have been deeply involved, and there are indications that the principle of objectively measuring how 'well' a patient feels is becoming more widely accepted amongst medical practitioners. On the other hand, however, the central concept of 'rationing' scarce resources in health care is still anathema to many doctors. They feel that they have an ethical responsibility to do whatever they believe to be best for the individual patient, regardless of its wider economic implications.

Nevertheless, there are encouraging signs that some leaders of the medical profession are starting to struggle with the ethical implications of a health care system in which there is a widening gap between what would be technically possible and what is actually affordable in practice. It is here that economists should be invited to become involved in these matters of medical ethics. Many of the issues referred to above need to be taken into account when deciding how best to allocate medical resources and what to say to the patient whose treatment is denied to him on economic rather than medical grounds.

At a more routine level, good data are essential for realistic economic analysis, and here both doctors and other health professionals, such as nurses, have a vital role to play. In the past there has sometimes been a trace of suspicion among doctors about the economists' true motives. This must be overcome, largely by educating doctors that their professional skills can be used to better advantage if they are guided by sound economic principles. Here the initiative lies with the economists to demonstrate more clearly the social value of their work. It is important to overcome the situation where doctors sometimes believe that cost-effectiveness studies of the cost-effectiveness studies themselves would disprove their value!

THE PROSPECT FOR CAREERS IN HEALTH ECONOMICS

Finally, on a totally optimistic note, it is clear from the chapters in this book that health economics is to become a growth industry. Albeit the growth is still from a very small base. In Britain with well over one million people employed in the National Health Service, there are probably fewer than one hundred health economists working in association with it, and only a handful actually employed directly by the Service.

When medical care is costing the taxpayer about £18 billion a year for the British National Health Service alone, in 1987 it is essential that the most effective use is made of such huge resources. Twenty-five years ago it was still naïvely assumed that doctors should be able to do everything which was technically possible for their patients. Now it is realised that that could never be the case, either within individual countries or worldwide. Indeed on the global scale the scope for the application of practical health economics is enormous, as Professor Brian Abel-Smith points out. But, echoing the last sentence of the previous section, 'quis custodiet?'; if health economists are to extend their activities they must clearly demonstrate their value in terms of improvements in the quality and distribution of medical care. The various contributions in this book strongly suggest that health economics indeed has a major role to play in improving the effectiveness of international health care in the next 25 years. Health economists have a responsibility to demonstrate the truth of this statement both to politicians and to doctors. If they can do so, the profession should gain well deserved recognition for its contribution to the well-being of mankind.

REFERENCES

Feldstein, M. (1967) *Economic analysis for health service efficiency.* North Holland, Amsterdam.
Maynard, A. and Ludbrook, A. (1981) 'Thirty years of fruitless endeavour?' in J. Van der Gaag and M. Perlman (eds) *Proceedings of the World Congress of Health Economics*, North Holland, Amsterdam.

Teeling Smith, G. (1984) *A new NHS act for 1996?* Office of Health Economics, London.

Ware, J.E. *et al*. (1986) 'Comparison of health outcomes at a Health Maintenance Organisation with those of fee-for-service care'. *Lancet*, i, 1017.

Part One

The International Scene

2

The Future of Health Economics in the UK

A.J. Culyer

A UK RESEARCH CONSENSUS?

What determines the selection of research topics by researchers? The question needs to be answered if one is to make an informed guess about future patterns of work. It may be proximate demand by researchers: that is, whatever currently takes their fancy. But in that case one naturally probes deeper to ask the determinants of their fancy: whether, for example, it is the attraction of solving problems that arise from within the discipline itself and that generate their own logical imperatives. (For example: why do individuals demand health care? Partly because they demand health. Why do they demand health? Partly because . . .) Or whether, instead, it is their perception of what fruits of research are most urgently needed in their community.

In either case, the research that is *actually* done cannot be determined by demand from researchers alone. Although the sort of research that can be done by a single scholar seated at his or her desk is partly immune from the compromising (as some would see them) influences of research sponsors, in the generality of cases it seems clear that the supply of research funds, reflecting the demands of research *sponsors*, must also play an important role in determining what gets done, if only for the compelling reason that funding is a *sine qua non* for doing the work.

Here evidently is a fruitful source of tension since it is not obvious that the research needs perceived from a disciplinary perspective, or those perceived to exist in society by practitioners of the discipline, will be coincident with those perceived by those with funding power. One might expect the divergences to be smaller the more closely knit the research community is itself (not least because

15

of the research proposal reviewing process that will tend to apply shared criteria of what is important). The more intimate and on-going the liaison between sponsors (research customers) and researchers (contractors) the fewer and less important the antagonisms between these groups are again likely to be (the charge may reasonably even be heard that one group has 'captured' the other, though who, whom, may often be hard to perceive!) Moreover, the more pluralism in both the research community and potential sponsors, the greater the variety to be expected in current and future research programmes, making the future accordingly the harder sensibly to foretell.

In the UK the health economics research community is rather closely knit. Its members know one another mostly on a first name basis. The twice yearly meetings of the Health Economists' Study Group together with its annual publication *HEART* (Parkin and Yule, various) which lists all members' research interests, have played an important role in the building of what seems to be a consensus on what the important research topics area. This consensus has been furthered by the existence in the UK of only three major concentrations of health economists: at York, Aberdeen and in the Economic Adviser's Office at the DHSS, of which only one has a training programme in graduate health economics, form-ing the prime origin of trained British personnel in the field. The demand-supply distinction is blurred significantly by the member-ship of the DHSS health economists in the HESG and their active involvement in it, so that any naïve supposition that the role of government health economists *vis-à-vis* those in the university and medical research communities is merely to represent governmental demands for research results is very wide of the mark. Moreover, although there is no monopoly of research funding in the UK, there are no fundamental substantial or methodological differences between the major funding agencies like the DHSS itself, the Nuffield Provincial Hospitals Trust, or the Rowntree Trust.

The UK health economics community is characterised — I conjecture largely because of the factors just discussed — by a thoroughgoing convergence. There is, as already stated, a widespread meeting of minds about which areas of work need the most attention. But there is also a widespread meeting of minds about the kind of methods to be used and there is also a widespread meeting of minds about the sort of assumptions it is reasonable to make. Before illustrating this multi-faceted convergence hypothesis I should say — lest anyone suppose otherwise — that although the consensus may be seen to be in some sense a mark of the success of health economics in the UK as 'coming of age', it is nevertheless an unhealthy state, for it encourages complacency, assumptions are taken for granted and left unexamined — or unre-examined. Focus is on 'normal science' and attention turns away from fundamental questioning of the roots of the discipline. I thus find myself on the one hand to be in the congenial position of sharing the presumptions of a consensus that I have helped to shape while, on the other, being in the less congenial position of suspecting that the victory represented in the consensus is a little too complete.

In one sense, the UK professional consensus makes forecasting easier. All one needs to do is to identify the types of issue that are likely to be in the future wind and one can then fairly readily extrapolate the sort of research response that there will be. For example, one may identify as an 'issue' the ageing of the population. The research response will be partly to examine closely the basis for such demographic forecasts, to warn against naïve health care cost extrapolations (for the obvious but nevertheless easily overlooked point that one of the reasons why people live longer is that they are healthier and often demand less health care), and to point out the *endogeneity* of health costs: for example the degree to which one institutionalises health care for the aged is not determined by their numbers, nor is the extent to which one adopts 'heroic' measures determined by the numbers in terminal care (as Robert Evans has pointedly asked in this context: who are the heroes? 1985, p. 447). From this the extension of attention to questions of effectiveness and cost-effectiveness is then natural and, I would guess, wholly predictable.

AN UNSTABLE EQUILIBRIUM?

While all that seems perfectly plain, I strongly suspect that the current consensus is actually a rather unstable equilibrium. The very fact that the consensus exists means that there are reputations to be made for those daring enough to depart from it. For a long while there has been, for example, a UK consensus about the general inappropriateness of market mechanisms in the production, distribution and finance of health services. The publication of a volume just at a time when it appeared this consensus might be threatened by political pressures (McLachlan and Maynard, 1982) was characteristic and devastatingly successful. Ranks closed. The agenda was

THE FUTURE OF HEALTH ECONOMICS

preserved. Consensus was affirmed. But there are contrary straws in the wind (for example Green, 1985; Minford, 1985, ch. 3) and powerful traditions elsewhere (especially in the USA) on which the dissenters may respectably draw. Who knows when these may burst out from the undergrowth with a major and effective challenge to the consensus, thoroughly confounding all one's predictions?

In what follows I shall, not knowing the laws that govern the motion of intellectual history, take the present consensus as given and assume — despite my doubts — that it will continue. The external forces that may affect future patterns of research (mainly from the research sponsors' side) will be taken to be extensions of existing trends: a fast pace of technological development, with swift diffusion; ageing population; and continuing political concern about value for money. Onto a description of the current pattern of health economics research and its distinctively British character can then be grafted a conjectured impact of these rather predictable trends.

CURRENT CURRENTS IN HEALTH ECONOMICS

Figure 2.1 displays the principal topics that are studied in health economics and is based on one that my colleagues and I at York (England) have found to be a useful framework within which to develop both graduate teaching and research programmes (Williams, 1986). It shows not only the principal topics (with at times somewhat arbitrary boundaries placed between them) but also the logical linkages between them, with the direction of the arrows indicating that the box from which a pipeline flows has contents which are for the most part logically prior to the contents of the box into which it flows. It is of course these systematic interlinkages that makes it possible to create a research programme that is more than merely a collection of topics.

Broadly speaking, the four central boxes, A, B, C, and D, contain the analytical 'engine room' of health economics while the four peripheral boxes E, F, G, and H, are the main empirical fields of application for whose sake the engine room exists. This, of course, is not to deny that, for some, boxes A, B, C, and D are of inherent substantive concern. Most health economists, however, would, I conjecture, treat the contents of these boxes as instrumental, needed not so much for their own sakes (despite the intellectual satisfaction to be had from limiting one's work to the topics to be found in them) as for the effective leverage that they enable one to

Figure 2.1: A schematic diagram of health economics

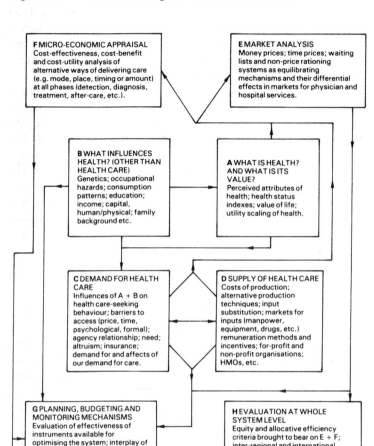

bring to bear on the policy issues contained in boxes E, F, G, and H.

For entirely conventional reasons, I want to begin with boxes C and D — demand and supply — rather than with the boxes that are, as you will see, logically prior. Moreover, I shall begin with box D. This contains the topics to be expected in supply-side economics: matters concerning the inputs with what may be seen as a kind of production function (or, in the language of Russell, 1983, a 'technology matrix'). What is being 'produced' is an issue taken up in connection with the discussion of box A. The illustrative references I shall draw on will no doubt reflect the prejudices of a British economist. I shall not, however, restrict them to British topics or authors. At times I shall say something about the differences between British and other foci of research interest.

The major topics in box D include the search for empirical forms that efficiently summarise often very complex relationships (the classic in this field is Feldstein, 1967); estimating the extent and type of substitution that may be possible between inputs (e.g. Feldstein, 1967 again for hospitals; Reinhardt, 1972 for general practice); comparing hospital costs (e.g. Coverdale, Gibbs and Nurse, 1980; Sloan, Feldman and Steinwald, 1983); computing marginal, as distinct from average, costs (e.g. Neuhauser and Lewicki, 1976); appropriate levels of hospital reimbursement and the ways hospitals respond to them (Romeo, Wagner and Lee, 1984; Russell, 1984; Sloan, 1984), the ways in which suppliers respond to different incentive packages, for example, hospital doctors' responses to budgetary incentives (e.g. Wickings and Coles, 1985) or fee for service and other methods of physician renumeration (e.g. Evans, 1972; Woodward and Warren-Boulton, 1984); effects of regulation on the supply industries (e.g. Cooper, 1966 or Scherer, 1985).

The health care 'industry' (Evans, 1984) is a complex supply network embracing not only the obvious sectors like hospitals and clinics (public and private) but also institutions operated by other authorities (e.g. some social services, some residential care for the elderly and for children) and also some at least of the main (usually private sector) suppliers of medicines and equipment, as well as independent agencies under contract (including GPs in the UK). As always, in defining an industry, there is some doubt about where it is best to draw a line between what is included and what excluded. The lines drawn in practice are really more a matter of convention than inferable from any sacred first principles to which all health economists would subscribe.

The complexity on the supply side derives largely from the

tremendous variety of institutions to be found around the world and the great variety of behavioural responses to different kinds of reward/penalty structures. On the demand side (box C), the complexity has a different source. There are grave dangers in simply carrying over the usual presumptions of economics into this territory. First, health care is not demanded for its own sake, and, indeed, one would rather not demand any at all. It is a *derived* demand: derived from an underlying current demand *for health* and from one's entire past history of demanding health (or not, as the case may be!). So one evidently cannot talk about the demand for health care without also considering the contents of boxes A and B, of which more anon (the pioneering perceptions here by an economist are in Arrow, 1963). Secondly, no man is an island. There is lots of evidence that one person's health, or health care consumption, is also of concern to others — not perhaps *all* others, but usually still lots. One reason for this is a risk of contagion or infection, but the reasons also go a good deal beyond that into the realm of 'fraternity' (Culyer and Simpson, 1980 is a review) that implies a demand concept that transcends the individual's demand for his or her own sake and that has important consequences for the type of finance of health care and the means by which it is channelled to suppliers. Thirdly, and in part growing out of these attributes, it is quite natural for people to talk the language of 'need', no matter how much it may catch in economists' throats (Culyer, Lavers and Williams, 1971), and so it has commanded some attention (Culyer, 1976; Williams, 1978). On the prevalent view, health care is a *necessary condition* (viz, 'needed') for the achievement of some (better) health state that the individual ought to be in. It thus clearly embodies two quite distinct concepts: one to do with the 'oughtness' of need (the question of the *entitlement* of an individual to the end state preferred which clearly involves making value judgements, including value judgements about value judgements, such as: who ought to be making these value judgements?) and the other to do with the *instrumentality* of health care as a means of accomplishing the desired end state, which is not, in contrast, a value question but an empirical one to do with which option (there is usually more than one) is more effective at bringing about the end state.

The importance of these sorts of issue for Box E will be self-evident, if only because the best worked out case for the use of market mechanisms is based upon the twin notions of demand as revealing individuals' own perceptions of their welfare (rather than 'need') and of the insigificance of third party effects. If these are denied, many conventional sequelae become highly suspect. You can also see, however, that box D is beginning to infiltrate itself into box C, because questions of *effectiveness* of health care belong in D as characteristics of production functions. But they also belong in Box C — does it make sense to say that someone 'needs' (or even 'ought to receive') *ineffective* health care? Ought I to be entitled to receive ineffective care at your expense? The answers to these questions seem obvious. But they are questions that hardly arise at all in other spheres of economics.

A further major complication on the demand side again occurs as the result of contaminating leaks from box D. The typical consumer of health care is unlike the typical consumer of most goods. He or she may feel sick, but will not usually know why, whether the feeling will go away on its own, how long it will last, what can be done to help it go away, what these actions will cost, or how effective, quick acting and permanent in result these various actions may be. For all these items of information, the patient relies on the doctor. The patient may often initiate an *episode* of care (Stoddart and Barker, 1981), but the demand for *treatments* is heavily influenced by the doctor acting presumably as an agent for the patient (Evans, Parish and Sully, 1973; Evans, 1974, 1976; Fuchs, 1978). This agency relationship is also found in other walks of (usually professional) life (Tuohy and Wolfson, 1977, 1978). So here we have the physician acting as both supplier and demander. The potential thereby afforded under different systems of physician payment and terms of service for physicians to be tempted away from a pure agency role will be apparent, but the extent and significance (for health or welfare) of 'supplier-induced demand' is much discussed in the literature (e.g. Pauly, 1980; Zweifel, 1981; Dionne and Contandriopoulos, 1985; Reinhardt, 1985; Ferguson, 1985) and shows no sign of diminishing for the foreseeable future.

Finally, the fact that health care can on occasion be extremely costly (costlier than an average family's entire wealth, let alone the wealth of the poor or the elderly who are usually more in need of health care than others) and the fact that one's need for it at any future date is usually uncertain, raise a whole set of issues to do with insurance, its comprehensiveness, subsidy and organisation, all of which can impact on demand and introduce new extensions in the scope of health care industry as well as raising issues that need to be considered in boxes G and H (reviews of health insurance issues include Rosett, 1976; Newhouse, 1978; Evans and Williamson, 1978; Maynard, 1982).

These considerations, both individually and as a group, render it quite inappropriate to make two commonplace assumptions in economics. One is the practical working assumption that demand and supply are independent of each other so that if, say, supply rises, one may assume that the (downward-sloping) demand curve will stay put and thereby unambiguously predict that quantity per period will rise and price will fall. That no longer becomes a reliable working assumption in health care markets. The other assumption is the value judgement to the effect that each individual knows his or her interest best and, moreover, has no interest in the interests of others. The choice of source of value in health economics thus becomes an issue that is far more frequently debated than in most other areas of economics.

One may also detect regional differences in prevailing opinion, with the views that supplier-induced demand is relatively insignificant and that doctors are sufficiently good agents for patients for the traditional welfare interpretation of demand to be sustained both being far more prevalent among health economists in the USA than in Canada, Europe or Australasia.

Moving backwards along the logical train we come to boxes A and B. These boxes are both to do with the demand for health from which the demand for health care is derived. First comes the concept of health itself — box A. This is one of the more multi-disciplinary areas in which you are likely to find economists, epidemiologists, operational researchers, psychologists and sociologists all working — and sometimes even working together (Culyer, 1983)! There have been major methodological breakthroughs in both concept and experimental technique drawing in a variety of intellectual sources: construction of health status indices (e.g. Hunt, McKenna and McEwen, 1981), health utility indices (Torrance, 1986), quality adjusted life-years (Kind, Rosser and Williams, 1982; Torrance and Zipursky, 1984; Williams, 1985) and related outcome measures reviewed in this volume by Alan Williams (see also OHE, 1985). Although such health measures do not explicitly *value* health outcomes, their use highlights the value judgements that are inherent in their construction (Culyer, Lavers and Williams, 1971; Culyer, 1978) as well as providing a range of new empirical techniques where until recently there were none. Similar claims can be made for the burgeoning literature on the valuation of life-saving or death-postponing events which is, today, far removed both conceptually and empirically from the early attempts to value life by treating people as though they were carthorses (see, for example, Mishan,

1971; Jones-Lee, 1976, 1982 and, for a dissenting view, Broome, 1978, 1985). The carthorse approach seems to be monopolised these days by medical writers.

Box B contains a variety of determinants of health, broadly genetic and environmental (for example Gravelle, 1984 on unemployment and health; Leu, 1984 on smoking and health). The principal economic contribution in this territory goes under the name 'human capital'. This is much more than a mere revamping of an earlier view about the value of a healthy life as the present value of an expected net income stream over an expected life time. Rather it represents a distinctive way of treating *health* itself: as a capital stock that depreciates and that can be invested in, whose demand influences and is influenced by the demand for other human investments (e.g. educational ones) and ties directly into other applied fields of economics — most obviously, labour economics (Grossman, 1972; Dowie, 1975; Phelps, 1976; Cropper, 1977; Fuchs, 1982; Muurinen, 1982). The core of this work concerns the interaction between a health production function and a health demand function and it is perhaps the most distinctively original corpus of thought in the health economics literature, drawing as it does on two of health economics' distinctive features (production theory and demand theory) and combining them in the rigorous language of capital theory to produce implications that ramify deeply into policy issues as apparently different as the prevention of infant mortality and the relationship between health and learning disabilities.

Boxes A, B, C, and D are the essential toolkit — what I earlier called the engine room. Boxes E, F, G, and H are mainly concerned with application. In those countries having explicit markets for health care, there is a rich set of phenomena to explain and market-improving devices to explore, many of which arise out of the special characteristics of the demand for health described above and from methods of finance (especially health insurance and modes of physician payment). Many of these markets have non-price rationing resulting from the operation of the insurance market, professional restraints and governmental regulations. Although non-money prices exist in such markets (e.g. time prices, see Acton, 1976) these acquire greater relative prominence in systems like the UK's that rely less on market allocation: time prices, distance prices (Russell, Akehurst, Glass and Reid, 1976) waiting time (Lindsay, 1980; Cullis and Jones, 1985; Iversen, 1986) and the analysis of the effects of this profusion of non-price allocation methods really deserves far more attention that it has so far received. Another under-tilled field within the general territory of box E is the behaviour of non-profit supply agencies which, though it has received some attention (e.g. Newhouse, 1971; Jacobs, 1974; Harris, 1977; Pauly, 1980; Muurinen, 1986) remains an important field in which there is still no consensus either about appropriate modelling approaches or about how non-profit agencies may be expected to respond to changes in the parameters that constrain their behaviour.

The questions in box E are both 'positive' (what actually happens, happened, or is predicted to happen) and 'normative' (evaluating better and worse ways of getting things done). Box F, by contrast, is almost entirely normative and takes one into the realm of cost-effectiveness (CEA) and cost-utility (CUA) and the cost-benefit analysis (CBA). The bulk of the work of British health economists is to be found here either in direct application or once removed in boxes A, B, C, and D on logically prior questions of principle that need resolution if they are to be successfully applied in box F. In CEA, the notion of output is usually unidimensional and the main focus is on cost (e.g. Rich, Glass and Selkon, 1976 on screening; Culyer and Maynard, 1981 on treating ulcers; Ludbrook, 1981 on renal disease; Lowson, Drummond and Bishop, 1981 on oxygen supplies). In CUA a more serious attempt is made to explore the nature of output more fully, drawing on the health index literature (e.g. Wright, Cairns and Snell, 1981; Fordyce, Mooney and Russell, 1981, on the care of the elderly; Buxton, Acheson, Caine, Gibson and O'Brien, 1985 on heart transplants; and Williams, 1985 on comparing several treatment and prevention programmes). CBA is the most ambitious kind of exercise of which few genuine formal published examples exist (but see Hagard, Carter and Milne, 1976 on spina bifida) though its methodology is being increasingly practised in the British regions and districts in routine option appraisals (see Akehurst and Buxton, 1985; Akehurst and Holtermann, 1985). The variation in quality of work in this field is immense (and much continues to be done without the participation of any trained economist). Fortunately, several guides to good practice exist (e.g. Williams, 1974b; Drummond, 1980, 1981; Culyer and Horisberger, 1983; Culyer, 1985). There is every reason to expect to see this sort of work continuing in all countries but especially, perhaps, those in which greater reliance is placed on planning mechanisms than markets. The quality of the empirical work is also rising — a happy trend that can also be expected to continue.

Box G is a relatively underdeveloped area as far as economics is concerned. On the one hand there is not enough recognition of the importance of including managers in the appraisals of box F, so that some work of that kind is still-born by virtue of having failed to spot the relevant options, weight the costs and benefits appropriately, or tackle explicitly the administrative and organisational aspects of change that can so easily serve to sabotage the best intentions (see e.g. Akehurst and Buxton, 1985; Culyer, 1985). On the other there is too little study of the planning, budgeting and monitoring mechanisms of the health care system. Although this is less true in the USA (see e.g. Luft, 1981; Enthoven, 1978; Welch, 1985) where a more pluralistic system encourages the emergence of new forms of organisation and where there is less consensus amongst health economists about the preferred general characteristics of the medical market, the typical British enterprise in this territory is either defensively conservative (e.g. McLachlan and Maynard, 1982) or rather modest (e.g. Wickings and Coles, 1985). This is notwithstanding some trenchant critiques of the distortions induced by present budgetary arrangements and the false incentives they provide (e.g. Williams, 1974a).

Box H is concerned with the highest level of appraisal: comparative system costs (e.g. Poullier, 1985, 1986); determinants of international expenditure differences (Kleiman, 1974; Newhouse, 1975, 1976; Maxwell, 1981; Evans, 1983; Leu, 1986) and outcome differences (Vayda, 1973; Culyer, Maynard and Williams, 1982). The genre is fraught with difficulties arising from differing accounting conventions, uncertain purchasing powers, widely differing cultures, barely comprehended technologies and production functions, highly imperfect aggregate health measures and the absence of widely agreed theories of the behavioural consequences of alternative modes of provision and finance. Progress in this territory is highly contingent on further work in *all* the preceding boxes. At present its main value is to refute the more naïve claims made for or against 'our' system which — as we all know — is the 'best in the world' and to debunk the self-interest that often masquerades as dispassionate analysis.

FUTURE CURRENTS IN HEALTH ECONOMICS

In most of the topics in the eight boxes of the chart it has to be said that the USA is the leader. The USA typically produces the very best and the very worst in health economics — as it does most other things. The British focus is fairly heavily concentrated on box F together with its associated prior topics in A and B (e.g. health measurements and the valuation of life) and C and D (e.g. production functions and need). Unless there is some fundamental change in the consensus about the general appropriateness of the NHS as a form of organisation there is little incentive for British health economists to follow their American colleagues with research into non-profit and for-profit institutions, health maintenance organisations, insurance systems and the like. To the extent that research engages with such issues, my guess is that it is much more likely to be as a kind of rearguard, defensive, action designed to refute — or even stifle — any nascent promarket developments.

The main foci for research that I foresee are therefore those that arise in response to trends or changes that occur within a basically static institutional framework. One of these trends has already been alluded to: effects of an ageing population. Others include continuing pressure for cost containment and fast developing and diffusing technological inventions, both of which would seem to entail increasing focus upon where it already is — box F. As has already been pointed out there is some linkage into box G from box F partly through the more comprehensive appraisals that I hope to see in the future that will take more explicit account of managerial consequences, and partly because the research programme into health outcomes and cost and production functions will increasingly yield up routine measures that can be used by managers to monitor the system and by controllers to monitor the performance of managers.

So we have seen the future. It is the present — only more so.

REFERENCES

Acton, J.P. (1976) 'Demand for health among the urban poor, with special emphasis on the role of time'. In Rosett, 1976.

Akehurst, R.L. and Buxton, M.J. (1985) 'Option appraisal in the NHS A Guide to Better Decision-making'. *Nuffield/York portfolio, no. 8*, Nuffield Provincial Hospitals Trust, London.

────── and Holtermann, S. (1985) 'Provision of decentralised mental illness series: an option appraisal'. *University of York Centre for Health Economics, Discussion Paper 5*, CHE, York.

Arrow, K.J. (1963) 'Uncertainty and the welfare economics of medical care'. *Am. Econ. Rev., 53*, 5, 941–73.

Broome, J. (1978) 'Trying to value a life'. *J. Pub. Econs., 9*, 91–100.

────── (1985) 'The economic value of life'. *Economica, 52*, 281–94.

Buxton, M.J., Acheson, R., Caine, N., Gibson, S. and O'Brien, B. (1985)

Costs and benefits of the heart transplant programmes at Harefield and Papworth hospitals. HMSO, London.

Cooper, M.H. (1966) *Prices and profits in the pharmaceutical industry.* Pergamon, London.

Coverdale, I., Gibbs, R. and Nurse, K. (1980) 'A hospital cost model for policy analysis'. *J. Opl. Res. Soc., 31,* 801–11.

Cropper, M.L. (1977) 'Health, investment in health, and occupational choice'. *J. Pol. Econ., 85,* 1273–94.

Cullis, J.G. and Jones, P.R. (1985) 'National Health Service waiting lists: a discussion of competing explanations and a policy proposal'. *J. Health Econs., 4,* 21, 119–35.

Culyer, A.J. (1976) *Need and the National Health Service.* Martin Robertson, Oxford.

—— (1978) 'Need, values and health status measurement'. In Culyer and Wright, 1978.

—— (ed.) (1983) *Health indicators: an international study for the European Science Foundation.* Martin Robertson, Oxford.

—— (1985) 'Health service efficiency: appraising the appraisers'. *University of York Centre for Health Economics, Discussion Paper 10,* CHE, York.

—— and Horisberger, B. (eds) (1983) *Economic and medical evaluations of health care technologies.* Springer, Berlin.

—— and Jönsson, B. (eds) (1986) *Public and private health services: complementarities and conflicts.* Basil Blackwell, Oxford.

—— Lavers, R.J. and Williams, A. (1971) 'Social indicators: health'. *Social Trends, 2,* 31–42.

—— and Maynard, A.K. (1981) 'Cost-effectiveness of duodenal ulcer treatment'. *Soc. Sci. and Med., 15C,* 3–11.

—— Maynard, A. and Williams, A. (1982) 'Alternative systems of health care provision: an essay on motes and beams'. In M. Olson (ed.) *A new approach to the economics of health care.* American Enterprise Institute, Washington.

—— and Simpson, H. (1980) 'Externality models and health: a Rueckblick over the last twenty years'. *Econ. Record, 56,* 222–30.

—— and Wright, K.G. (1978) *Economic aspects of health services.* Martin Robertson, Oxford.

Dionne, G. and Contrandriopoulos, A-P. (1985) 'Doctors and their workshops; a review article'. *J. Health Econs., 4,* 1, 21–34.

Dowie, J. (1975) 'The portfolio approach to health behaviour'. *Soc. Sci. and Med., 9,* 619–31.

Drummond, M.F. (1980) *Principles of economic appraisal in health care.* Oxford University Press, Oxford.

—— (1981) *Studies in economic appraisal in health care.* Oxford University Press, Oxford.

Enthoven, A. (1978) 'Consumer-choice health plan'. *New Eng. J. Med., 298,* 650–3, 709–20.

Evans, R. (1972) *Price formation in the market for physician services in Canada 1957–1969.* Prices and Incomes Commission, Information Ottawa, Canada.

—— (1974) 'Supplier-induced demand: some empirical evidence and

28

implications'. In M. Perlman (ed.) *The economics of health and medical care*. Macmillan, London.
—— (1976) 'Modelling the economic objectives of the physician'. In R.D. Fraser (ed.) *Health economics symposium: proceedings of the First Canadian Conference*, Queen's University Industrial Relations Centre, Kingston.
—— (1983) 'Health care in Canada: patterns of funding and regulation'. *J. Health Politics, Policy and Law*, 8, 1, 1–43.
—— (1984) *Strained mercy: the economics of Canadian health care*. Butterworths, Toronto.
—— (1985) 'Illusions of necessity: evading responsibility for choice in health care'. *J. Health Politics, Policy and Law*, 10, 3, 439–67.
—— Parish, E.M.A. and Sully, F. (1973) 'Medical productivity, scale effects, and demand generation'. *Can. J. Econs.*, 6, 3, 376–93.
—— and Williamson, M.F. (1978) *Extending Canadian health insurance: options for pharmacare and denticare*. University of Toronto Press, Toronto.
Feldstein, M.S. (1967) *Economic analysis in health service efficiency*. North-Holland, Amsterdam.
Ferguson, B.S. (1985) 'Physician objectives and resource allocation'. *J. Health Econs.*, 4, 1, 35–42.
Fordyce, J.D., Mooney, G.H. and Russell, E.M. (1981) 'Economic analysis in health care 2: an application to care of the elderly'. *Health Bull.*, 39, 1, 29–38.
Fuchs, V.R. (1978) 'The supply of surgeons and the demand for operations'. *J. Hum. Resources*, 8, Supp., 35–56.
Fuchs, V.R. (1982) 'Time preferences and health: an exploratory study'. In V.R. Fuchs (ed.) *Economic aspects of health*. University of Chicago Press for the National Bureau of Economic Research, Chicago.
Gravelle, H.S.E. (1984) 'Time series analysis of mortality and unemployment'. *J. Health Econs.*, 3, 3, 297–306.
Green, D.G. (1985) 'Which doctor? A critical analysis of the professional barriers to competition in health care'. *Research Monograph 40*, Institute of Economic Affairs, London.
Grossman, M. (1972) *The demand for health: a theoretical and empirical investigation*. Columbia University Press for the National Bureau of Economic Research, New York.
Hagard, S., Carter, R. and Milne, R.G. (1976) 'Screening for spina bifida cystica: a cost-benefit analysis'. *Brit. J. Prev. Soc. Med.*, 30, 40–53.
Harris, J. (1977) 'The internal organization of hospitals: some economic implications'. *Bell J. Econs.*, 8, 21, 467–82.
Hunt, S.M., McKenna, S.P. and McEwen, J. (1981) *The Nottingham health profile: Manual*. Mimeo, University of Nottingham.
Iversen, T. (1986) 'An interaction model of public and private health services: surgical waiting lists'. In Culyer and Jönsson, 1986.
Jacobs, P. (1974) 'A survey of economic models of hospitals'. *Inquiry, 11*, 2, 83–97.
Jones-Lee, M.W. (1976) *The value of life: an economic analysis*. Martin Robertson, Oxford.
—— (ed.) (1982) *The value of life and safety*. North-Holland, Amsterdam.

29

Kind, P., Rosser, R. and Williams, A. (1982) 'Valuation of quality of life: some psychometric evidence'. In Jones-Lee, 1982.
Kleiman, E. (1974) 'The determinants of national outlay on health'. In M. Perlman (ed.) *The economics of health and medical care*. Macmillan, London.
Leu, R.E. (1984) 'Anti-smoking publicity, taxation, and the demand for cigarettes'. *J. Health Econs., 3*, 2, 101–16.
—— (1986) 'The public-private mix and international health care costs'. In Culyer and Jonsson, 1986.
Lindsay, C.M. (1980) *National health issues: the British experience*. Hoffman-La Roche, Nutley.
Lowson, K.V., Drummond, M.F. and Bishop, J.M. (1981) 'Costing new services: long-term domicilary oxygen therapy'. *Lancet*, i, 1146–9.
Ludbrook, A. (1981) 'A cost-effectiveness analysis of the treatment of chronic renal failure'. *Appl. Econs., 13*, 337–50.
Luft, H.S. (1981) *Health maintenance organizations: dimensions of performance*. Wiley, New York.
McLachlan, G. and Maynard, A. (eds) (1982) *The public private mix: the relevance and effects of change*. Nuffield Provincial Hospitals Trust, London.
Maxwell, R.J. (1981) *Health and wealth*. Lexington Books for Sandoz Institute, Lexington.
Maynard, A.K. (1982) 'The private sector in Britain'. In McLachlan and Maynard, 1982.
Minford, P. (1985) *Unemployment: cause and cure* 2nd edn. Basil Blackwell, Oxford.
Mishan, E.J. (1971) 'Evaluation of life and limb: a theoretical approach'. *J. Pol. Econ., 79*, 687–705.
Muurinen, J-M. (1982) 'Demand for health: a generalised Grossman model'. *J. Health Econs., 1*, 1, 5–28.
—— (1986) 'Modelling nonprofit firms in medicine'. In Culyer and Jönsson, 1986.
Neuhauser, D. and Lewicki, A.M. (1976) 'National health insurance and the sixth stool guiac'. *Policy Analysis, 2*, 2, 179–96.
Newhouse, J.P. (1971) 'Toward a theory of nonprofit institutions: an economic model of a hospital'. *Am. Ec. Rev., 60*, 1, 64–74.
—— (1975) 'Development and allocation of medical care resources: medico-economic approach'. In *Development and allocations of medical care resources*. 29th World Medical Assembly, Tokyo.
—— (1976) 'Medical care expenditure: a cross-national survey'. *J. Hum. Res., 12*, 115–25.
—— (1978) *The economics of medical care*. Addison-Wesley, Reading, Mass.
Office of Health Economics (1985) *Measurement of Health*. OHE, London.
Parkin, D. and Yule, B. (eds) (various) *Health economists' activities, research and teaching* (HEART). CHE, University of York.
Pauly, M.V. (1980) *Doctors and their workshops: economic models and physician behavior*. University of Chicago Press, Chicago.
Phelps, C.E. (1976) 'Demand for reimbursement insurance'. In Rosett, 1976.

Poullier, J-P. (1985) *Measuring health care 1960–1983*. OECD, Paris.
—— (1986) 'Levels and trends in the public-private mix of the industrialized countries' health systems'. In Culyer and Jönsson, 1986.
Reinhardt, U.E. (1972) 'A production function for physicians' services'. *Rev. of Econs and Stats., 54*, 55–66.
—— (1985) 'The theory of physician-induced demand: reflections after a decade'. *J. Health Econs., 4*, 2, 187–94.
Rich, G., Glass, N.J. and Selkon, J.B. (1976) 'Cost-effectiveness of two methods of screening for asymptomatic bacteriuria'. *Brit. J. Prev. Soc. Med., 30*, 54–9.
Romeo, A.A., Wagner, J.L. and Lee, R.H. (1984) 'Prospective reimbursement and the diffusion of new technologies in hospitals'. *J. Health Econs., 3*, 1, 1–24.
Rosett, R.N. (ed.) (1976) *The role of health insurance in the health services sector*. National Bureau of Economic Research, New York.
Russell, I. (1983) 'The evaluation of computerized tomography: a review of research methods'. In Culyer and Horisberger, 1983.
—— Akehurst, R., Glass, N.J. and Reid, N. (1976) 'Cost-benefit analysis in health services research: a case study of the location of ambulatory care'. *Procs. Am. Stats. Assoc.* (Soc. Stats Section), 167–72.
Russell, L.B. (1984) 'Prospective reimbursement and new hospital services'. *J. Health Econs., 3*, 1, 77–82.
Scherer, F.M. (1985) 'Post-patent barriers to entry in the pharmaceutical industry'. *J. Health Econs., 4*, 1, 83–8.
Sloan, F.A. (1984) 'Hospital rate review: a theory and an empirical review'. *J. Health Econs., 3*, 1, 83–6.
—— Feldman, R.D. and Steinwald, A.B. (1983) 'Effects of teaching on hospital costs'. *J. Health Econs., 2*, 1–28.
Stoddart, G.L. and Barker, M.L. (1981) 'Analyses of demand and utilization through episodes of medical service'. In Van der Gaag and Perlman, 1981.
Torrance, G.W. (1986) 'Measurement of health utilities for economic appraisal'. *J. Health Econs., 5*, 1–30.
—— and Zipursky, M.D. (1984) 'Cost-effectiveness of antepartum prevention of Rh immunization'. *Clins. in Perinatology, 11*, 2, 267–81.
Tuohy, C.J. and Wolfson, A.D. (1977) 'The political economy of professionalism: a perspective'. In M.J. Trebilcock (ed.) *Four aspects of professionalism*. Consumer Research Council, Dept. of Consumer and Corporate Affairs, Ottawa.
—— and Wolfson, A.D. (1978) 'Self-regulation: who qualifies?' In P. Slayton and M.J. Trebilcock (eds) *The professions and public policy*. University of Toronto Press, Toronto.
Van Der Gaag, J. and Perlman, M. (eds) (1981) *Health, economics and health economics*. North-Holland, Amsterdam.
Vayda, E. (1973) 'A comparison of surgical rates in Canada and England and Wales'. *New Eng. J. Med., 20*, 1224–6.
Welch, W.P. (1985) 'Health care utilization in HMOs'. *J. Health Econs., 4*, 4, 293–308.
Wickings, I. and Coles, J. (1985) 'The ethical imperative of clinical

budgeting'. *Nuffield/York portfolios, no. 10*, Nuffield Provincial Hospitals Trust, London.

Williams, A. (1974a) 'The budget as a (mis)information system'. In A.J. Culyer (ed.) *Economic policies and social goals: aspects of public choice*. Martin Robertson, Oxford.

———— (1974b) 'The cost-benefit approach'. *Brit. Med. Bull., 30*, 3, 252–6.

———— (1978) '"Need": an economic exegesis'. In Culyer and Wright, 1978.

———— (1985) 'The economics of coronary artery bypass grafting'. *Brit. Med. J., 291*, 326–9.

———— (1986) 'Health economics: the cheerful face of the dismal science?' Forthcoming presidential address to Section F of the British Association.

Woodward, R.S. and Warren-Boulton, F. (1984) 'Considering the effects of financial incentives and professional ethics on "appropriate" medical care'. *J. Health Econs., 3*, 3, 223–38.

Wright, R.G., Cairns, J.A. and Snell, M.C. (1981) *Costing care: the costs of alternative patterns of care for the elderly*. Sheffield University Joint Unit for Social Services Research, Sheffield.

Zweifel, P. (1981) 'Supplier-induced demand in a model of physician behaviour'. In Van Der Gaag and Perlman, 1981.

3

The Development of Health Economics in Europe: Problems and Prospects

Simone Sandier

The evolution of health economics in Europe over the years ahead will be determined by developments in the discipline to date as well as the prospects for health care systems from technical, social and economic perspectives. Both of these considerations contain quantitative and qualitative elements, the former relating, for example, to the numbers of research workers and studies as well as the levels of finance and the latter linked to the countries of study, the institutions involved, the themes investigated and the nature of health care organisation. It is not possible to discuss all these aspects comprehensively in the present chapter; instead a few examples will be employed to illustrate some of the points at issue.

Since the end of the Second World War European nations have been directing an increasing proportion of their human, technical and financial resources towards the health sector, reflecting growing economic prosperity, the public's desire for enhanced levels of well-being, progress in diagnostic techniques and care and the general availability of social protection in the field of sickness. These factors are of course in reality interlinked, both causes and consequences of each other, although the precise influence of each has yet to be convincingly demonstrated.

The establishment of collective systems of financial protection, covering all or part of the expenditure on medical consumption, has greatly contributed towards an awareness of how the cost of this consumption has grown, and to the formulation of questions which have become classic subjects of study and research for health economists. The following are examples of this:

How much is spent on health care, who benefits from this expenditure, who finances it, what rewards accrue to which producers, what factors influence change?

How effective are the different methods of allocating resources in terms of their health, economic and social implications, how are geographical and social class disparities reduced? Which method contributes more, or at lower cost, towards improving the health care indicators?

It could be said that the teams working in the area of health economics in various European countries have been developed in order to respond to these types of questions and, with this objective in mind, have evolved a range of techniques for observation and analysis, taking into account both the general characteristics of health care and the organisational peculiarities of providing and financing health care in their own countries.

International bodies like the World Health Organization (WHO), the OECD and the EEC have made a substantial contribution towards increasing awareness in Europe of the economic problems connected with the health care sector. It may be argued that by organising working parties, publishing studies, consulting regularly with national governments in order to carry out comparative studies, these organisations have progressively urged countries which had not already done so to start evaluating the resources made available to the health care sector and to take a critical look at the efficiency of their health care systems.

This supportive role will continue to play a part in the future and, provided current work continues, it may be anticipated that health economics studies will also be developed in southern European countries, which were slower in coming to this discipline than their northern neighbours. In this way studies carried out in West Germany, Belgium, France, Italy, the Netherlands and Switzerland should be further supplemented by those carried out in universities and under the auspices of national or local governments in Spain, Portugal and Greece. These new teams will have to prove their originality and dynamic approach in the choice of subjects they tackle and in disseminating their results: in this way their work should reinforce European strengths in this field and help to make studies carried out in Europe stand out from those carried out in North America in a very different economic, political and social climate.

In fact the subjects chosen for health economics research in a particular country are largely determined by financial considerations. Resources are usually provided by government or private groups who hope to be able to draw from the results of these studies, stimulating new ideas which will enlighten decision-making in the short, medium or long term. Even now, research projects in the area of health economics have far more chance of being accepted in practice if they take account of political and social realities and are concerned with real problems actually facing any given country. It seems likely that the diminishing availability of research grants that is presently accompanying the decline in economic growth will reinforce this trend. It is therefore with an increasing awareness of the political, economic, demographic, cultural, health and social environments of their own countries that health economists in Europe will have to approach the general themes that are preoccupying decision-makers everywhere as far as expanding and diversifying the health-care sector is concerned.

More particularly, national economic studies will have to take account of the various measures adopted by different European states at different times to meet the financial risks connected with sickness: a public insurance system financed by contributions or a national health system financed from the state budget, or even a mixed system combining the public and private sectors in varying proportions. These measures constitute the guiding principles for controlling the health care system of each country: politically it is easier to modify some of them whilst conserving the underlying principles than to exchange them for a completely new approach. The difficulties encountered in Italy in setting up a National Health Service illustrate this point.

Financiers will therefore call upon health economists to analyse the relationships between the level and development of health care consumption on the one hand, and the practical aspects of financing health care systems on the other: advance payment of costs by patients or direct payment of producers by insurance schemes, reimbursement rates which vary according to the type of care or the patients, the methods of reimbursing health care expenditures, the size of budgets and the way in which they are allocated at a national or regional level. One research theme naturally connected with the above is the possible impact of social protection, which seeks to control health care expenditure, on one of the principal objectives of social policy: equal access to excellent medical care for all sections of the community.

The interactions between the health care sector and demography and the general economic situation provide health economists with a source of study which is still relatively untapped. Three areas might be mentioned by way of illustration:

The ageing population in Europe, due mainly to the declining birth rate and, to a lesser extent, to increased life-spans, is often considered to be a factor that will accelerate health care expenditure. Studies must be carried out to confirm or invalidate this proposition and to show how the system of distributing care can be adapted to demographic change.

Ageing populations, even if studies showed that they would not necessarily entail a marked acceleration in medical consumption, give rise to economic and financial problems similar to and connected with those posed by retirement pensions with regard to their deleterious impact on obligatory contributions. In many countries, where sickness insurance resources comes from employees' and employers' contributions, the redistribution of resources associated with the collective financing of medical consumption will increasingly tend to reflect sympathy between different generations, or between those in work and those out of work. Health economists will have to analyse the consequences of the fact that an increasing proportion of the fruits of labour will be spent on a non-productive sector; they will also have to investigate which systems of finance are best suited to this new reality.

Economists will have to examine comprehensively the contribution of the health care sector to economic life in general, a subject which has yet to be extensively analysed. In many countries it has been pointed out that the health care sector has created employment both directly and indirectly as a result of certain industrial activities, although exact figures have not always been available. Studies should be carried out to clarify these points and to go even further in measuring the possible productivity gains linked to improved health. The answers could usefully illuminate the debate regarding the appropriate level of a country's resources that should be devoted to medical care.

It should be possible for research in the field of health economics in Europe to continue to expand into new areas if the groups currently working in this area obtain the support necessary to their development. This implies not only making financial resources available, but also providing a range of other conditions appropriate to effective work: the existence of an appropriate institutional framework, access to good basic statistical information etc. In this respect Europe, and in particular continental Europe, is dragging its feet.

The statistical data which constitute the basic prerequisite for economic analyses in the area of health care are still insufficient in many countries. Progress in this respect, which depends mainly, but not exclusively, on government, lies not only with statisticians, but with health economists as well, who could play a useful part in defining the parameters to be measured based on their relevance to the country's health care planning. Depending on the country, statistics could be acquired from a number of sources, from scrutinising administrative and financial documents to the results of detailed surveys. In European countries the existence of social protection agencies is especially advantageous, since they can gather information regarding medical consumption and the behaviour of health care suppliers from a large number of individuals or companies distributed throughout the country. The measures adopted to meet the costs of, and the methods of remunerating, the producers have a direct influence on the scope and detail of the information that can be collected.

These statistics are relatively economical to gather as a by-product of the activities of the agencies which finance health care and pay the producers: for this reason they can be obtained at regular intervals. It is to be hoped that in the future this type of information will be more systematically exploited and interpreted in all European countries so as to provide a basis for annual assessments of national health care accounts, tracing the flow of finance between the suppliers, the consumers and the bodies financing medical care. However, for understandable reasons of confidentiality, it is unlikely that insurance bodies will provide economists with all of the information they require in order to carry out their analyses. In many cases special surveys aimed at analysing particular issues will have to be undertaken by interviewing the public or medical organisations; this is often the case with in-depth studies of a sample population, with cost-benefit analyses of specific medical actions, and with research which has to use a mass of information relating both to the medical sector and other aspects of social life.

In common with their colleagues throughout the world, European health economists have available to them a wide spectrum of analytic tools ranging from descriptive statistics to sophisticated modelling techniques. In any event the design and choice of suitable indicators is a very important preliminary step which often determines the quality of the results. These indicators must have real significance not only at the economic level, but also at the medical and social level: moreover, they must be susceptible to objective measurement and comparison in different settings and over time. In practice, research is mainly financed by the public sector, and to a lesser extent by the pharmaceutical industry or other private groups. There is little reason for this situation to change: on the contrary, there is every reason to believe that, in total, the funds available for health economics studies will not grow as rapidly as the health care sector itself; but in fact a rapid increase in health expenditure might justify an equivalent rise in funds available for health economics research. It is even conceivable that budgetary limitations and the constraints they impose might modify the current distribution of health economics studies to the benefit of specialised services within central or regional governments, with the difficulties faced by private or public research centres and universities increasing accordingly.

Indeed, external bodies are often the first to shoulder the burden of the budgetary rigours imposed on ministries or other administrations. The number of research contracts awarded in many European countries, and yet more so the sums devoted to them, have already tended to decline. This situation is often accompanied by increased demands not only for scientific quality, which would be acceptable, but also for administration evidence such as detailed accounts, which discourages or even diverts some excellent research workers towards other activities.

This background of constraints, whether deplorable or not, nevertheless represents a reality which will influence the diversity and the number of research projects undertaken. In this situation research workers are going to have to prove their originality and will have to resist two ready solutions: simply transposing the work of their North American colleagues to the European situation and bowing to political pressures within their own countries.

In the field of health economics, as in many other spheres, the influence of the United States is very strong: some European research workers have in fact been trained in North American universities, many journals of health economics are of American origin and in the United States sufficient resources have been available to permit excellent, highly varied studies to be carried out which provide prestigious points of reference for Europeans. The presence of many leading Americans at international conferences also contributes to the dissemination of the American influence in Europe.

Thus in recent years fashionable topics in the United States, such as 'deregulation' or 'competitive markets' have become the focus of research interest in many European countries and national vocabul'iries have had to assimilate American abbreviations like 'HMO', 'DRG', 'PPO'. It is likely that in years to come health economists will also be inspired by other concepts originating in the United States, the country of innovation and experimentation. It is to be hoped that they will then be analysed critically, not forgetting that a US approach to a given problem may not be suitable for Europe, and may even represent a retrogressive step in certain European situations. It will be difficult for research workers in the field of health economics in Europe to eschew the characteristic approach of American studies if, as is natural, they seek the international recognition of their peers. It is to be hoped, however, that university courses in health economics will be developed in Europe and that, despite linguistic difficulties, European journals, conferences and research personnel exchange, will facilitate the dissemination of studies carried out in each country as well as the development of common methodologies suited to the health care problems and the socio-economic conditions of Europe. International bodies within Europe have a role to play in this context.

In theory planners, or more generally those responsible for the financing and distribution of care, would like to be helped in making their choices and to be able to justify them by reference to objective studies of health economics. In practice their decisions are taken within the framework of a complex spectrum of constraints, and they can find themselves in conflict with the results of such studies. During difficult periods governments, the principal source of study finance, often tend to look less at the quality of research than at its financial implications, or the obstacles that research findings might pose for the implementation of their policies, and this can result in additional constraints for research workers: taboo subjects, the withholding of statistics, checks and delays imposed on the publication of results. Research workers, depending on their reputation, their affiliations, their status, their immediate or long term ambitions, are more or less equipped to react to this type of financial and political pressure. The small number of research workers in health economics in Europe does, however, make them more vulnerable than their American colleagues: it restricts the number of studies they can carry out and reduces their ability to counter opposition to their findings.

Some research workers will be unaware of the pressures and will perhaps reap the benefits of this in the long term. Others will use their energies in elaborating sophisticated models which will remain theoretical for want of the basic statistical information indispensable to their practical application, and which will not therefore emerge as results that may be of use to planners. Others will avoid subjects which are too 'hot' or will present their results in such a way that they can only be used with difficulty outside scientific circles.

It has only been possible to give a brief picture of the work awaiting health economists in Europe over the next few years and the problems they will have to overcome in order to forge their identity. Furthermore, this description has necessarily been both global and partial at the same time. The situation is not uniform throughout Europe; it varies according to each country's social and political organisation: one factor in particular which determines the financing and subjects of health economics studies is the way in which the responsibility for health care planning is distributed between central government and regional authorities.

The list of research topics for the next few years goes well beyond that presented here: it comprises analyses of the health and economic consequences of technical progress, the wider application of cost-benefit analysis to different treatments, research into the respective roles of community and hospital medicine and many more.

The benefits of exchange between colleagues from different European countries should lead in the future to a common pursuit of health economics studies with an international flavour. This will involve, for example, collaborating in the collection of basic information from various countries. It will also embrace comparative studies of the different health care systems in existence, focusing especially on their successes and their weak points, with the experience of each serving to draw social policies in Europe closer together.

4

Health Economics in the Nordic Countries: Prospects for the Future

Bengt Jönsson

INTRODUCTION

When in 1979 an annotated bibliography of health economics was published in Sweden, Jönsson and Ståhl (1979), it included only 121 references despite a very generous interpretation of the sources. In the other Nordic countries, Denmark, Finland, Iceland and Norway, the number of publications on health economics was even fewer (see Griffiths, Rigoni, Tacier and Prescott, 1980). If the same criteria for inclusion in a bibliography of health economics had been applied today, less than ten years later, it would probably include over a thousand references. This shows that health economics is a very new, but rapidly developing, subject in the Nordic countries.

Before 1980 the concept 'health economics' was only known to and used by a small number of economists, who had learned about this field of applied economics through scientific journals, conferences and personal contacts with colleagues in the UK and USA. The establishment of the Group for Health Services Research in Oslo in 1976, the Swedish Institute for Health Economics (IHE) in 1979, the economics unit within the Swedish Planning and Rationalisation Institute of Health Services (SPRI) some years later and the Laboratory for Research in Community Medicine and Health Economics (now the Department of Health Economics and Public Health) at Odense University in 1980 denote a change. It was recognised by various parties, the pharmaceutical industry (IHE), the providers of health services (SPRI), the medical research councils (Oslo) and universities (Odense) that health economics research could make a contribution to the improvement of health services and that resources for such research had to be created. In Finland no specific institution was created but a number of economists went to

41

York University for training in health economics, funded by the Yrjö Jahnsson Foundation. In 1980 the first meeting of the Nordic Health Economists' Study Group was held in Sweden. Since then this group has met annually alternating between the Nordic countries.

The establishment of the above mentioned research centres made health economics research more multidisciplinary and more focused on practical application. A number of studies were published showing that health economics and health economists could be used to address important questions in health policy. This has created a fast growing interest among clinicians, administrators, health planners and politicians to learn more about and apply the concepts, theories and results of health economics. Diffusion into the health care system has slowly begun, almost exactly 20 years after 'modern' health economics was introduced as an academic discipline. However, health economics is still generally unknown to the general public.

HEALTH ECONOMICS AND THE NORDIC HEALTH CARE SYSTEMS

Health economics as a topic is closely related to how the economic problems in health care are perceived and defined. The goals, structure, financing and development of the health care system determine the aim and direction of health economics in each country. In order to understand the development of health economics in the Nordic countries it is important to know some facts about the health care systems and their economic development in the different countries.

Despite adverse economic developments during the last decade the Nordic countries are among the wealthiest in the world. GDP *per capita* averaged almost $13,100 in 1980. Twenty-two million people shared almost $300 billion total GDP in 1980 or 8.5 per cent of GDP in OECD Europe. Health care expenditure *per capita* is also among the highest in the world (see Table 4.1). The share of GDP spent on health care varies from 6.6. per cent in Finland to 9.2 per cent in Sweden. Note that statistics based on national accounts principles underestimate health care expenditure in Denmark and Norway.

The economic stagnation after the first oil crisis affected the health care sector after a significant lag. Between 1975 and 1980 the share of health expenditure in GDP increased in all Nordic countries, while after that it has remained constant or decreased. The

Table 4.1: Health care expenditures in the Nordic countries in 1982

Country	Share in GDP (%)	US$ per head	Public expenditure	% of resources spent in publicly owned institutions
Denmark	6.8	746	90	71
Finland	6.6	692	79	72
Iceland	7.6	865	87	
Norway	6.8	930	87	67
Sweden	9.7	1168	91	90

Source: OECD (1985), Rohde (1986).

significant reduction in the annual real growth rate of total health expenditure has highlighted that resources for health care are scarce and that continued development of health care in Scandinavia and Finland presuppose improved efficiency. The hope that health economics can contribute in this respect is a major factor behind the growing interest in health economics as a tool in health policy making.

Health care is mainly financed through taxation. Public insurance is a major financial source for non-institutionalised care and for dental care and medicines. Private insurance is nearly non-existent and direct charges to the consumer very small. The public monopoly of financing makes cost containment technically easy but politically difficult. It also nearly eliminates the possibility of undertaking empirical studies of different financing mechanisms in health care. This makes it difficult to apply a significant part of health economics research in the USA to the situation in the Nordic countries. However, another important aspect of the health care systems in the Nordic countries is regionalisation. This is most profound in Sweden and Denmark where financing is based on local (county and municipal) taxation. The growing research on health maintenance organisations (HMOs) can be relevant in formulating alternatives to the present system.

Characteristic of the Nordic countries is the high share of resources spent in public institutions. Competition between providers plays a very limited role in resource allocation in health care. Physicians working within hospitals are generally paid on a salary basis. In Sweden this is also the case for physicians in ambulatory care, for pharmacists and for a significant number of dentists. It is thus understandable that one will find very little research about health manpower economics in health care in Scandinavia. Studies by Rohde (1982) and Nygaard (1984) are exceptions to the rule.

Research that aims to improve planning and administrative decisions dominates. In this respect there is a similarity between the UK and the Nordic countries, and British health economists, predominantly from the University of York, have played a significant role in advising Nordic health economists how health economics can be used in a public health system. One example is the economics of waiting lists (see Iversen, 1986).

The opportunities for studies of the effects of alternative financing mechanisms and economic incentives in health care are limited. The empirical data are simply not there. Another data problem is lack of reliable cost data for use in productivity and cost-benefit studies. Budgeting and accounting data are mainly related to institutions on a very high level of aggregation. It is very difficult to obtain data on the resources used for specific programmes or groups of patients. One consequence of this is that health economists have to spend a lot of energy doing rather trivial calculations of costs related to specific technologies and diseases. Since such calculations are time-consuming and expensive, less resources are left for tackling more interesting problems of calculating indirect costs and measurement of outcome. However, significant improvements in health care information systems are under way which will facilitate economic calculations. It has been a tiresome but necessary step in the development of health economics to point out the need for this change.

TRENDS IN HEALTH ECONOMICS RESEARCH

Health care expenditure analyses have so far formed the major part of health economics research in the Nordic countries. Both the factors behind the rapid expansion of health services 1960–75 and the deceleration during the last decade have been thoroughly investigated. For a survey of the Swedish studies, see Ståhl (1981) and for Denmark, see Pedersen and Petersen (1979). Since cost containment does not pose a serious problem this type of study disappeared as the rapid growth of health expenditure came to an end. The long-term relation between the growth of health care expenditure and economic growth has been generally accepted. However, controversy still persists about how the increasing number of elderly will affect future health care expenditure.

The focus has shifted to studies of the determinants of productivity and ways and means to increase this. For examples see Lindgren and Roos (1985), Jönsson and Rehnberg (1985), Indenrigsministeriet (1986) and Sintonen (1986). This research follows two different directions. The first aims at improving planning and administration within the present structure of the systems. Clinical (frame) budgets, diagnosis-related groupings and patient-based internal cost accounting are key concepts in this strategy. The second aims at introducing more markets, incentives and competition in order to improve efficiency (see Ståhl, 1981). Studies of the private/public mix in health care will be a major interest for health economists in the years to come, see Culyer and Jönsson (1986) and Rohde (1986). Hopefully the regionalisation of health care in the Nordic countries will allow for some experimentation as a basis for empirical analysis. A key question will be how efficiency and equity can be combined.

In public health care systems, where resources are allocated through planning and administrative decisions, there is great scope for cost-benefit and cost-effectiveness studies to assist decision making. It is therefore not surprising that economic appraisal is one of the major fields of health economics in the Nordic countries, most notably so in Sweden. If we include cost-of-illness studies, which are closely related, this becomes even more apparent. Most academic dissertations in health economics fall into this category, for example Mattsson (1968), Jönsson (1976), Uhde (1977), Egon Jonsson (1980), Lindgren (1981) and Sintonen (1981). In the future cost-benefit, cost-utility and cost-effectiveness analysis will remain one of the major fields of health economics in the Nordic countries. Under the epithet 'medical technology assessment' economic appraisal is gaining wide acceptance among both clinicians and politicians. Special committees have been established in all the Nordic countries to promote an increased use of medical technology assessment as an aid in clinical decision making and health policy. The concept 'medical technology assessment' is wider than economic appraisal and includes, for example, ethical dimensions, but the contribution from health economics is essential and health economists will undoubtedly play a leading role in the development of this field. This is the field in which the Nordic countries are most likely to make a significant contribution. Clinical research in the

Nordic countries is very advanced, one example being clinical drug trials and, if health economics can be amalgamated with this research tradition, it can be a very fruitful combination. The establishment of the Centre for Medical Technology Assessment (CMT) in Linköping and the evaluation of the extra-corporeal shockwave lithotriptor for treatment of kidney stones are examples of how multidisciplinary research has been organised and conducted along these lines.

Another field in which Scandinavian and Finnish health economists can make significant contributions in the future is the social and economic determinants of health. Epidemiological research has a long tradition, high standard and unique data bases in the Nordic countries. So far epidemiologists and health economists have worked independently but a closer co-operation, from the time when studies are planned, can prove very beneficial for both parties. Odense University has been the main centre for epidemiological and survey-based health economics research. Over the years the health economists there have conducted extensive epidemiological studies, as a basis for studies of the demand for health (see Bentzen, Christiansen and Pedersen, 1985). The work by Søgaard (1983) on the relation between unemployment and health should also be mentioned. In Norway, a study of the economics of preventing tuberculosis using a sophisticated epidemiological model was published very early on (see Waaler, 1975). Later a study on treatment of hypertension, Waaler et al. (1978), integrated health economic aspects with original epidemiological analysis. In Finland and Sweden there are a significant number of health economists with an interest in and knowledge of epidemiology. This is an important resource for the future that can be utilised if the research councils make sure that a health economist is included as a full member of the research team when epidemiological studies are funded.

One particular area where economics and epidemiology can fruitfully be combined is the evaluation of primary prevention. The Nordic countries have been in the forefront in adopting 'health for all', the WHO philosophy for health policy, which emphasises prevention as a strategy for better health. A number of important epidemiological studies on which this strategy is based have been done in the Nordic countries. Now there is a need for careful evaluation of the projects implemented and health economics can make a significant contribution in studies of the goals, outcome, cost-effectiveness and distributional consequences of preventive programmes.

Health economics research in the Nordic countries has been empirically oriented. The theoretical contributions have been few. The main explanation for this is probably that the very few health economists there are have felt it necessary to work in most areas of the subject instead of specialising. Much has also been done to develop and market the subject and demonstrate the practical use of health economics. However, some contributions of a theoretical nature can be identified. Ståhl has published extensively on issues related to public choice and the 'voucher system' (Ståhl, 1980, 1981). Niels C. Petersen has also done theoretical research from a public choice perspective (Petersen, 1986), but his main research has been on demand for health (Petersen, 1984). Also J.-M. Muurinen (1982) has made contributions to the development of demand-for-health models. Methodological problems related to cost-benefit analysis in health care are addressed in some early dissertations (Jönsson, 1976; Uhde, 1977 and Sintonen, 1981). Lately the incentives generated by work environment policy measures have been investigated in a dissertation by Lyttkens (1985). The balance between theoretical and empirical research within health economics in the Nordic countries is probably not different from that found in other fields of economics. However, there are some reasons for concern which will be discussed later.

HEALTH ECONOMICS AS AN ACADEMIC DISCIPLINE

Health economics is defined by Culyer (1981) as the application of the discipline and tools of economics to the subject matter of health. If we accept this definition it implies that economists and departments of economics must play a leading role in the development of health economics. If we look back, we see this is what happened. In Sweden, the department of economics at the University of Lund, under the leadership of Professor Ingemar Ståhl, was the major centre for health economics during the 1970s. Research in health economics was a natural element in the department's broader specialisation in public economics. In Denmark, Kjeld Möller Pedersen and Terkel Christiansen, two economists from the department of public finance and policy at Odense University, were instrumental in introducing health economics. In Norway, the first major contribution was made by Aina Uhde, from the department of economics at the University of Bergen. In Finland, Harri Sintonen, although a civil servant within the Ministry of Health at that time, must be classified as a professional health economist. His training at the University of York and his dissertation at the department of social policy, University of Helsinki, makes this evident.

However, the economists were not the only actors on the stage. A number of persons with a background in medicine or health administration made significant contributions. Professor Finn Kamper-Jörgensen, a physician and now director of the Danish Institute for Clinical Epidemiology was the author of several papers on the economics of screening and road accidents in the early 1970s. His textbook, Kamper-Jörgensen (1974), is still one of the most important publications in health economics in Scandinavia. Peter Hjort, a professor of medicine, took the initiative with the Group for Health Service Research within the Norwegian Medical Research Council and included health economics as a major part of the group's research programme. He has been the leader of the research group from its start. In Sweden, Professors Björn Smedby and Egon Jonsson, using their affiliations with the Medical Research Council and SPRI respectively, have made great efforts to introduce health economics.

Obviously there has been some tension between those who approached health economics as a discipline and those who started with health economics as a topic, 'the economy' of health care. Looking at health economics as a topic, it is of course correct to stress that health economics is multidisciplinary and that disciplines other than economics, for example medicine, ethics, political science and sociology, can make important contributions to the understanding of the processes and institutions that govern the allocation of resources to health care. What has been more difficult for economists to accept are statements that, for a variety of reasons, economics is not relevant or suitable for application to matters of health. One example that is frequently put forward is the concept of discounting. Instead, it has been proposed, there is a need to develop a 'new' economics for use in economic studies of health matters.

Part of the tension can be explained by misunderstandings on both sides. Persons involved in health care often have a biased and incomplete view of economics as a discipline assuming that economics is only about money. Economists have frequently misunderstood the health problems they have studied or for other reasons provided a biased study and not used the best methodology. Part of the tension is of course explained by the fact that different interests are involved and it has on the whole been very productive. It has forced economists to improve their practice in health economic studies and health professionals to learn more about economics as a discipline. Perhaps the most important step forward during the last ten years has been the development of the co-operation between economists, health professionals and other scientists in studies of the economic problems of health care. The institutional framework in the Nordic countries has helped stimulate such co-operation. The leading academic research centres like the Department of Health and Society and the Centre for Medical Technology Assessment, University of Linköping, the Institute for Health Economics and Prevention at the University of Odense and the Group for Health Science Research in Oslo are multidisciplinary. The Swedish Institute for Health Economics (IHE), through its relation to the pharmaceutical industry, has a close link to the health services and to clinical research. The four Nordic 'planning institutes', SPRI in Sweden, DSI in Denmark, NIS in Norway and the Finnish Hospital League are part of the health care system in each country.

A special link between health economics and the medical faculties has been established through the system of adjunct professors. Björn Lindgren (IHE) and Egon Jonsson (SPRI) in Sweden hold appointments in the faculty of medicine at the university and there is a similar arrangement with the faculty of medicine in Oslo, Norway. Even if these positions are part-time and temporary, they provide important links between economics and medicine and are a basis for future development.

The existence of several competent and well established multidisciplinary research centres in Scandinavia makes the future for the development of health economics as a topic bright indeed. In Finland, the future development is still mainly linked to the activities of a few persons. It is more questionable what will happen with the development of health economics as a discipline. Will these centres be strong enough to foster theoretical development or will their research mainly be of an empirical and applied character? A key question is what will happen to health economics within university departments of economics. So far most economists trained in the field of health economics have left the university departments for a continued research career in other institutions. To my knowledge there is currently no senior economist mainly working on health economics in an economics department in the Nordic countries. There are several explanations for this. There has been a shift from micro- to macro-economics, including monetary economics and banking, over the last ten years. The total number of professors with an interest in public economics has been reduced. University departments in Scandinavia and Finland are small, which makes specialisation difficult. If economic research was concentrated in fewer, bigger departments it would be easier to include one health economist as part of the faculty.

The future development of health economics in the Nordic countries would clearly benefit if a major research programme for health economics research were established at one or two university departments of economics under the leadership of a full professor. However, there are mechanisms that can at least partly compensate for the lack of this. Two chairs in health economics have been established so far, one at Linköping University in 1981 and one at Odense University in 1985. These chairs, though not formally in the departments of economics, create opportunities for research and research education in health economics. The PhD-programme in Linköping now includes about ten economists. In Lund there is a close collaboration between IHE and the department of economics which makes it possible to recruit and educate economists for research in health economics. Since health economics is developing rapidly internationally there is also a scientific network that makes it possible to follow and participate in the progress of this sub-discipline without being part of the scientific community of professional economists.

It is a safe guess that the schools of medicine will increase their engagement in health economics and that we will see appointments of full professors of health economics at the major faculties of medicine in the future. Health economics is already introduced as part of the medical curriculum in most schools. Earlier experience with statisticians and sociologists has shown that the integration of other disciplines into medical research and education is not that easy and a great deal of thought must be given to how this should best be done.

HEALTH ECONOMICS AND HEALTH POLICY

Has health economics had an impact on health policy in Scandinavia and Finland so far? It is very difficult to answer this question because of the difficulty of detecting such an influence. It is easier to identify some areas where health economists have been asked for advice directly. The most obvious example is vaccination programmes, for which a number of cost-benefit studies have been undertaken in all the Nordic countries (see, for example, Pedersen *et al.*, 1985). The impact of these studies on policy has probably been small due to a number of factors. Many studies have been undertaken *ex post facto*, after the introduction of the vaccination programme. A number of studies have suffered from great methodological deficiencies, both from an economic and an epidemiological viewpoint. The lack of co-operation between economists and epidemiologists has been fatal for the studies. One extraordinary exception is the study by Pedersen *et al.* (1985). This study was initiated by the National Board of Health and the Ministry of the Interior *before* a decision to introduce mass vaccination against measles, mumps and rubella and was done by a research team of epidemiologists, clinicians and an economist. A decision was made to include these vaccinations in the law about free vaccination from 1 January 1987. Without the cost-benefit study it would probably have been difficult to convince the government to finance this programme. Another study that is generally judged as influential on policy is Waaler *et al.* (1978) on the costs and benefits of hypertension treatment strategies. It had a profound effect on the management of hypertension in Norwegian primary health care.

Lack of impact on policy does not necessarily mean that there are defects in the economic analysis. Very often decision makers in health care lack incentives to make their choices according to social costs and benefits. Instead they are interested in a narrower range of (financial) benefits and costs. The policy decision can also be influenced by factors that are difficult to account for in economic analysis. A study in Sweden (Ernst Jonsson, 1980) showed very clear net benefits from water fluoridation. Concern about unknown side-effects and ethical arguments made the Swedish Parliament decide not to introduce this preventive measure. It can of course be argued that an economic analysis should include all possible effects but in practice there will always be some effects that only the decision maker himself can bring into the verdict. Finally, one should also remember that an economic analysis is only one among several inputs to a decision process.

Another area where health economists have been asked to give policy advice is dental care (Sintonen, Maljonen, Heinonen and Myntsinen, 1983; Sintonen, 1986; Jönsson, Faresjö and Westerberg, 1983). These studies are concentrated on the balance between public and private dental care but the research projects have been broadened and the economics of dental care will probably be a major research field within health economics in the future. The policy implications are of an indirect nature and impossible to detect.

Since health economics research in the Nordic countries has been empirical and policy-oriented it has probably had an influence on policy but this should not be exaggerated. However, health economics still lacks influence in major policy areas like medical technology, health manpower, health planning and health management. So far no major impact can be seen but the future could be different.

In the field of medical technology assessment a number of new processes and institutions have been created that can give economic appraisal the same position in health care as in most other industries. This does not necessarily mean a large number of health economists within the health service. The major work has to be done by the health professionals themselves. In the future doctors will become interested and active in the economic appraisal of medical technologies. The introduction of cost-effectiveness as a new criterion for registration of new medicines has been discussed in Sweden. Even if this does not become law, it is reasonable to assume that health economics will be of great importance in the evaluation of drugs and in reimbursement policy in the future. In Denmark an office of health economics has been created within the Department of the Interior. Health economists are also regularly used as advisers within the National Board of Health. In Sweden, a health economist has been appointed to the National Board of Health and Welfare. In Norway one of the leading health economists serves as adviser within the Ministry of Health. In Finland, several health economists work in the Ministry of Social Affairs and Health on research and planning and the National Board of Health has recently published a booklet on the major topics for future health economics research (Pekurinen, 1985). This demonstrates an increasing demand for health economists and great expectations about what health economics can contribute. Are these expectations realistic? There are a lot of examples of misunderstanding about the contribution health economics can make. The time has come to make a serious study of this as a basis for developing the dialogue between demand and supply. Health economics and health economists can make a contribution to health policy but maybe not in the way most policy makers believe. It will take a long time to explain that health economics neither starts nor ends with cost accounting.

CONCLUSION

Twenty years have passed since the publication by Speek (1966) of the first major health economics paper in the Nordic countries. This can be seen as the start of health economics, although there are earlier contributions, for example Groundstroem (1914) and Rydenfelt (1949), in the tradition of Dublin and Lotka and Petty. During the first ten years, the development was slow and merely academic. Important contacts were established with health economists in the USA and UK, primarily at the University of York. At the end of the 1970s a number of important research centres were established in Denmark, Norway and Sweden and in Finland the Yrjö Jahnsson Foundation funded a number of scholarships for training in health economics at the University of York. This boosted development and resulted in a number of studies and publications showing that health economics could contribute to the understanding and solution of problems in the allocation of resources for health.

The development of health economics in the Nordic countries is closely related to local circumstances and institutions and the need for collaboration between economists, epidemiologists and clinicians has been recognised. A development and deepening of this collaboration can provide a basis for important contributions in areas like demand for health, evaluation of primary prevention and medical technology assessment.

The major weakness in the present development is the tendency towards separation of health economics from the economics departments at the universities. This separation reduces the opportunities for novel applications of the discipline of economics to the topic of health. The establishment of the Nordic health economists' study group and the close international contacts that Nordic health economists have developed can partly compensate for this. It is important that health economics does not lose its roots in the rapid development towards practical application and policy relevance.

ACKNOWLEDGEMENT

I am grateful for comments from Björn Lindgren, Kjeld Möller Pedersen, Finn Kamper-Jörgensen, Harri Sintonen and Hans Waaler.

REFERENCES

Bentzen, N., Christiansen, T. and Pedersen, K.M. (1985) 'Measurement of health status in a general population survey; choice of instrument; issues in scaling'. *Department of Public Finance and Policy, Occasional Papers no. 19,* Odense University.

Culyer, A.J. (1981) 'Health, economics and health economics'. In V. Van der Gaag and M. Perlman (eds) *Health, economics and health economics.* North-Holland, Amsterdam, New York, Oxford, pp. 3–11.

—— and Jönsson, B. (1986) *Public and private health services — complementarities and conflicts.* Basil Blackwell, Oxford.

Griffiths, D.A.T., Rigoni, R., Tacier, P. and Prescott, N.M. (1980) *An annotated bibliography of health economics — western European sources.* Martin Robertson, Oxford.

Groundstroem, E. (1914) 'Hammastaudit katsottuina kansantaloudelliselta kannalta' (Dental diseases from the viewpoint of national economy). *Proceedings of the Finnish Dental Society,* no. 13, 3–13.

Indenrigsministeriet (1986) Standardomkostninger og produktivitet for 96 somatiske sygehuse. En studierapport fra Indenrigsministeriet. Köpenhamn

Iversen, T. (1986) 'An interaction model of public and private health services: surgical waiting lists'. In Culyer and Jönsson (eds), *Public and private health services — complementarities and conflicts.* Basil Blackwell, Oxford.

Jönsson, B. (1976) 'Cost-benefit analysis in public health and medical care'. *Lund economic studies,* no. 12, Lund.

—— Faresjö, T. and Westerberg, I. (1983) 'Produktivitet i privat och offentlig tandvård'. *Rapport till expertgruppen för studier i offentlig ekonomi.* DsFi 1983:27, Stockholm.

—— and Rehnberg, C. (1986) 'Effektivare sjukvård genom bättre ekonomistyrning. *Rapport till expertgruppen för studier i offentlig ekonomi.* DsFi 1986:3, Stockholm.

—— and Ståhl, I. (1979) *Hälso — och sjukvårdsekonomi i Sverige — en bibliografi.* Liber Läromedel, Lund.

Jonsson, Egon (1980) *Studies in health economics.* Liber Tryck, Stockholm.

Jonsson, Ernst (1980) *Lönar det sig att tillsätta flour i dricksvattnet? En samhällsekonomisk utvärdering för perioden 1981–2025.* SOU. Liber förlag, Stockholm.

Kamper-Jorgenson, F. (1974) *Sundkitsokonomie: med socialmedicinski.* Institute of Social Medicine publication no. 3, University of Copenhagen.

Lindgren, B. (1981) *Cost of illness in Sweden 1964–75.* Liber, Lund.

—— and Roos, P. (1985) 'Produktionskostnads — och produktivitetsutveckling inom offentligt bedriven hälso — och sjukvård 1960–1980'. *Rapport till expertgruppen för studier i offentlig ekonomi.* DsFi 1985:3, Stockholm.

Lyttkens, C.H. (1985) 'Swedish work environment policy. An economic analysis'. *Lund economic studies,* no. 37, Lund.

Mattsson, B. (1968) 'Vägtrafikolyckornas samhällsekonomiska kostnader'.

Statens Trafiksäkerhetsråd, Rapport no. 116, Stockholm.

Muurinen, J.-M. (1982) 'Demand for health. A generalized Grossman model'. *Journal of Health Economics, 1*, 5–28.

Nygaard, E. (1984) 'Legers takstbruk — bestkrivelse og analyse'. *Gruppe for helsetjensteforskning. Rapport no. 3*, Oslo.

OECD (1985) 'Measuring Health Care 1960–1983'. *Social Policy Studies, 2*, Paris.

Pedersen, K.M. and Petersen, J.H. (1979) *Hvorfor kan den offentlige sektor ikke styres?* Berlingske Leksikon, Copenhagen.

—— Kauper-Jorgensen, F., Bjerregaard, P., Koch, C., Wagner, A.L. and Zoffman, H. (1985) 'An economic appraisal of a proposal for vaccination against measles, mumps and rubella'. *Department of Public Finance and Policy, Occasional papers no. 20*, Odense University.

Pekurinen, M. (1985) *Terveystalonstiede ja tutkimus (Health economics and research)*. National Board of Health Publications, no. 64, Helsinki.

Petersen, Niels C. (1984) 'Demand for health and demand for preventive and curative cure'. Laboratoriet for samfundsmedicinsk og sundhetsekonomisk forskning, *Rapportserien no. 6*, Odense Universitet.

—— (1986) 'A public choice analysis of parallel public-private provision of health care'. In Culyer and Jönsson (eds) *Public and private health services — complementarities and conflicts*. Basil Blackwell, Oxford.

Rohde, T. (1982) 'Lönninger ved sjukehus. Avtaleverk og lönnsutvikling 1979–81'. *Gruppe for helsetjensteforskning, Rapport no. 3*, Oslo.

—— (ed.) (1986) 'Privat og offentlig innsats i Nordens helsevesen'. *Gruppe for helsetjensteforskning, Rapport no. 3*, Oslo.

Rydenfelt, S. (1949) 'Vad kostar sjukdomarna vårt samhälle'. *Landstingets tidskrift, 36*, 129–139.

Sintonen, H. (1981) 'An approach to economic evaluation of actions for health'. *Official statistics of Finland, special social studies XXXII: 74*. Ministry of Social Affairs and Health, Helsinki.

—— (1986) 'Comparing the productivity of public and private dentistry'. In Culyer and Jönsson (eds) *Public and private health services — complementarities and conflicts*. Basil Blackwell, Oxford.

—— Maljonen, T., Heinonen, M. and Myntsinen, A. (1983) 'Economics of Finnish dental care'. *Official statistics of Finland, Special social studies*. Ministry of Social Affairs and Health, Helsinki.

Sögaard, J. (1983) 'Socio-economic change and mortality: a multivariate coherency analysis of Danish time series'. In J. John *et al.* (eds) *Influence of economic instability on health*. Proceedings, Berlin, pp. 85–112.

Speek, J.-E. (1966) Samhällsekonomiska och sociala aspekter på sjukvården. Sjukvårdsplan för Göteberg. Bilaga 2. Stadskontor, Götebergs. For an English translation of the basic ideas see Speek (1972).

—— (1972) 'On the economic analysis of health and medical care in a Swedish health district'. In M.M. Hauser (ed.) *The economics of medical care*. University of York, *Studies in economics no. 7*, George Allen and Unwin, London.

Ståhl, I. (1980) 'The growth of health care: two model solutions'. In Heidenheimer and Elvander (eds) *The shaping of the Swedish health system*. Croom Helm, London.

—————— (1981) 'Can equality and efficiency be combined? The experience of the planned Swedish health care system'. In M. Olson (ed.) *A new approach to the economics of health care*. American Enterprise Institute, Washington, DC.

Uhde, A.L. (1977) 'On the optimal allocation of resources to health care: implications for cost-benefit analysis'. *University of Bergen*, economic papers, no. 1, Bergen.

Waaler, H.T. (1975) *The use of dynamic models in the epidemiology of tuberculosis*. Universitetsforlagets Trykningscentral, Oslo.

—————— Helgeland, A., Hjort, P.F., Lund-Johansen, P., Lund-Larsen, P., Mathisen, R. and Storm-Mathisen, H. (1978) 'Höyt blodtrykk: Behandlingsprogram utbytte, kostnader'. NAVF/GHF, *Report no. 5*.

5

The Health Care Economy in the USA

Alain Enthoven

I propose to offer a perspective on the structure of the US health care economy from the early 1930s to the early 1980s, how it is changing in the mid-1980s, and where present trends seem likely to take us by the year 2000.

WHERE WE WERE: THE OPEN ENDED ERA

For fifty years, health insurance in the United States was based on 'free choice of provider', or what Charles Weller called 'guild free choice' (Weller, 1984). Every insurance plan was required to leave the patient completely free and unbiased in choice of doctor or hospital; every doctor in the community was able to participate in every financing plan on equal terms. This 'freedom' is not in the Bill of Rights. It is a medical-economic concept designed to prevent cost-consciousness on the demand side of the market for health care services. The insured patient was not cost-conscious. And the payer had no bargaining power because it could not direct patients away from costly providers without violating their freedom of choice. It created what Martin Feldstein characterised as 'permanent excess demand' for physicians' services (Feldstein, 1970), a sort of 'economic gravity-free space'. This cost-unconscious demand was combined with fee-for-service payment of physicians and fee-for-service or cost reimbursement for hospitals, which pay providers more for doing more, whether or not more is necessary or beneficial to the patient. Among other things, this economic model led to a very costly standard of care. Also it led to a predominant ethic that the doctor must do everything that might help the patient, cost not considered. This is a logical consequence of respect for patients'

57

preferences and is made possible by their comprehensive insurance.

Physicians were cohesive and politically powerful. They were able to enforce the 'guild free choice' model through coercive tactics such as boycotts of non-conforming insurance plans and denial of referrals, hospital admitting privileges and medical society member-ships to non-conforming doctors, and by influencing legislation. Physicians practised with a very wide range of professional autonomy, under very little peer or social control. There were very wide variations in practice patterns from one community to another (Wennberg and Gittelsohn, 1973). There was virtually no quality control or systematic peer review with serious sanctions. Because of 'permanent excess demand', physicians were quite free to practise in the specialties and locations they preferred, minimally influenced by patient needs.

Hospitals competed for doctors in a cost-unconscious market. They did this by offering technology and amenities, which led to ever more costly standards of care. Hospitals faced virtually no financial risk in their investment decisions. Because of 'guild free choice' and cost-reimbursement, they always had cost-unconscious payers to pay the cost of excess capacity. They did not have to compete for contracts with cost-conscious insurance plans. As a result, in the mid-1980s, we have twice the acute beds we need.

Government, responding to provider interests, ratified and rein-forced the 'guild free choice' model through the federal Medicare and Medicaid laws and through insurance laws prohibiting selective contracting in many states. Government subsidies to health care and health insurance were largely in the form of open-ended subsidies to the marginal cost of care, in the mistaken belief that those who spend more need more. That is, if a doctor and patient covered by Medicare or Medicaid agreed on a more costly rather than less costly treatment, government was likely to pay all or most of the extra cost. If employers and employees in an upper income group decided that the next $100 increment in pay should be in the form of health care benefits rather than cash, the full amount could be applied toward untaxed health benefits and the government would lose the $40 or $50 in income and payroll taxes that it would have received if the employees had been paid in cash. So these public policies biased private choices in favour of more costly care and more comprehen-sive insurance coverage.

Employers kept hands off. They were uninvolved and unin-formed. They focused on benefit package design (what services should be covered and what share of the cost should be paid by the patient) and financing questions without examining patterns of care. As late as 1981, one study found that 'corporations were neither greatly concerned nor strongly motivated to do much about their health benefit costs' (Sapolsky, Altman, Greene and Moore, 1981). Impelled by the tax laws, competition for employees, or collective bargaining, employers offered increasingly comprehensive insurance.

Insurance companies increasingly became passive financial intermediaries with a diminishing role. In the earlier years, Blue Cross and Blue Shield, provider-sponsored non-profit insurance companies, practised community rating, that is the same price was charged for the same benefits, regardless of group. Commercial insurance companies entered and offered experience-rated insurance, that is premiums tailored with increasing precision to the specific costs of each employment group. In the 1970s, the larger employers shifted to 'self insuring'. They decided to pay the medical bills of employees directly, and to hire insurance companies merely to advise them on structuring benefit packages, and to process claims, that is to review the doctors' and hospitals' bills and prepare a cheque drawn on the employer's bank account.

The consequence of all this was a very large and rapid increase in spending on health care. National health spending grew from $27 billion (5.3 per cent of the Gross National Product (GNP)) in 1960, to $355 billion (10.7 per cent of GNP) in 1983. Real *per capita* spending nearly tripled in 20 years. Private health insurance premiums increased from 13 per cent of pretax corporate profits in 1960 to 49 per cent in 1983. At this size, this growth rate in spending could not continue.

WHERE WE ARE NOW: IN RAPID TRANSITION

In the mid-1980s, the open-ended era is coming to an end. We are in transition from 'guild free choice' to 'market free choice'. That is, consumers are gaining the freedom to contract in advance with a limited set of providers (doctors and hospitals), voluntarily, usually for a year at a time, in exchange for what they perceive to be better benefits and/or lower cost. Central to this concept is the 'Competitive Medical Plan' (CMP) or 'limited provider plan' that links insurance and a limited set of providers so that the insurance premium reflects the ability of those providers to control cost. This divides providers into separate economic units which compete on

59

price as well as quality of care and service.

The 'product' is changing from many individual services the buyer could not possibly understand and control (picture a patient or an employee benefit manager trying to argue with the attending physician over the need for tests or procedures), to global units of care that can be shopped for, compared and priced in advance. We are changing to price per case and *per capita*. Clinical and financial information is being linked so that 'products' can be compared in terms of price and quality. Price competition is coming fast.

Why is this happening? A number of important factors came together to force the change. 'Guild free choice' medical care got too costly for government and employers. A *taxpayer revolt* started in California in 1978 with the passage of Proposition 13, a drastic tax-cutting referendum. Taxes were a major issue in the 1980 and 1984 national elections, and tax rates have been reduced sharply. At the same time, defence spending, which had declined from 8.3 per cent of GNP in 1970 to 5 per cent in 1980, providing room for growth in social programmes, reversed its decline, and reached 6.5 per cent of GNP in 1985. The federal government had to act to curtail growth in its health care outlays.

In 1982, *employers* were hard pressed by a recession, a strong dollar, an unfavourable trade balance, and high interest rates. Health spending jumped from 9.4 per cent of GNP in 1980 to 10.5 per cent in 1982. On top of that, employers came to fear that if they stayed on the open-ended system as government limited its outlays, providers would simply pass on to them the costs they could no longer recover from the government. So employers were motivated to act decisively. And the high rate of unemployment created an economic and psychological climate conducive to reductions in employee benefits.

In the 1970s, employers and government favoured price controls and other economic regulation to restrain health costs. But the 1970s proved to be a decade of regulatory failure in health care. Price controls, certificate-of-need laws regulating hospital investments, and Professional Standards Review Organisations attempting to control Medicare and Medicaid utilisation had little or no effect in limiting growth in aggregate outlays. Hospital price controls in several states had some effect, but not nearly enough to solve the problem. Research on public utility regulation showed it often protected producers, created hidden subsidies for groups not obviously meritorious and raised costs to consumers. By the end of the decade, regulatory approaches were pretty much discredited.

In the early 1970s, health policy thinkers were almost unanimous in the belief that market forces had no useful role to play in health insurance and health care services. The first serious challenge to this view came in 1970 when Paul Ellwood, Walter McClure and associates proposed a 'health maintenance strategy' leading to a diversified, pluralistic and competitive 'health maintenance industry' that would be largely self-regulatory and make its own investment decisions in the context of market forces (Ellwood, Anderson, Billings, Carlson, Hoagberg and McClure, 1971). Their proposal led to the Health Maintenance Organization (HMO) Act of 1973, a federal law providing subsidies to new non-profit HMOs and requiring employers to offer them to employees as an alternative to traditional insurance. In 1972 and 1973, Scott Fleming designed and recommended to the Nixon Administration a proposal he called 'Structured Competition in the Private Sector' (Fleming, 1973). It is a mark of the regulatory mentality of the times that even this market-oriented Republican Administration was not able to comprehend and appreciate Fleming's radical proposal. In 1977, while serving as a consultant to Secretary Califano in the Carter Administration, I designed and recommended an extension and elaboration of Ellwood, McClure and Fleming's ideas in the form of 'Consumer Choice Health Plan', a national health insurance proposal based on regulated competition in the private sector (Enthoven, 1978). Clark Havighurst criticised existing arrangements from the perspective of anti-trust law and made pro-competitive proposals (Havighurst, 1978). By the end of the 1970s, the idea of a price-competitive health care economy had attained intellectual respectability and a significant following in Congress.

In the early 1980s, membership growth in Health Maintenance Organizations (HMOs) and other Competitive Medical Plans (CMPs) began to accelerate. (An HMO provides comprehensive medical care services for a periodic payment, set in advance, that is independent of the patient's use of services. This is usually referred to as 'per capita prepayment' or 'capitation'.) Geographic spread elevated their status from a West Coast curiosity to a credible threat to the traditional system. HMOs began to attract significant private capital. Some not-for-profit firms converted to for-profit status. By the early 1980s, there were several national HMO firms with the capital, management systems and know-how that could enable them to enter new areas with assurance of success. Many non-randomised studies had found that HMOs could deliver comprehensive care for 10 to 40 per cent less than the open-ended fee-for-service sector

(Luft, 1978). In 1984, the RAND Corporation published the results of a randomised comparison showing that an HMO cut costs some 25 per cent compared to fee-for-service, which helped to put to rest concerns that apparent cost reductions by HMOs were merely the result of favourable risk selection. The demonstrated practical success of HMOs added to the credibility of the competitive idea.

Finally, the power of *organised medicine* to block competition broke down under the combined weight of several forces. In 1975 the Supreme Court ruled that the 'learned professions' were subject to the anti-trust laws. Anti-trust actions by federal and state government agencies followed. The increasing supply of doctors meant that adherence to 'guild free choice' principles could no longer assure newly-trained doctors an opportunity for a good living. The incentive to break ranks and contract with a CMP as a way of securing patients increased sharply. With the growth in importance of specialties, academic medicine and HMOs, physicians identified their interests more narrowly and not with organised medicine as a whole. And finally, the growth in costs inspired the development of countervailing political power in the form of employer and employer-labour coalitions.

Impelled by these fiscal pressures, *government* broke out of the restraints of the 'guild free choice' system and began to limit its outlays for health care. In 1981, Congress allowed departures from the 'freedom of choice' provision in Medicaid and allowed states to engage in selective contracting with providers for negotiated prices for services to Medicaid beneficiaries. (Medicaid is a joint federal-state programme that pays for the medical care of poor aged, blind, disabled people and poor families with dependent children.) Coupled with this, the Congress reduced the federal share of Medicaid. By the mid-1980s, many states were experimenting with various types of CMP and 'managed care' schemes to serve Medicaid beneficiaries.

In 1982, Congress imposed effective limits on the growth in Medicare reimbursement per hospital inpatient case. (Medicare is the federal insurance programme for the aged and disabled.) Cost per case would not be allowed to grow faster than a price index of inputs hospitals buy plus one per cent. In 1982, Congress also enacted an 'HMO CMP option' in Medicare, a *per capita* basis of payment that allows Medicare beneficiaries who choose HMOs to obtain more comprehensive coverage by subscribing to an economical health care organisation. The payments are related to what each beneficiary would have cost Medicare if he or she had remained in the fee-for-service sector. There is much in the HMO model that is likely to appeal to many Medicare beneficiaries: especially lower cost, freedom from the complex paperwork in Medicare reimbursement, financial predictability and organisation of comprehensive services. Ultimately, this is likely to become the health care delivery system of choice for most Medicare beneficiaries.

At the same time, state governments moved to facilitate competition. In 1982, acting under pressure from an employer-labour coalition, the California legislature overturned the prohibition on selective contracting with providers by health insurance companies, and authorised them to negotiate with providers and pass the savings on to the insureds. The states of Illinois and Michigan followed. The new laws authorise what is known as Preferred Provider Insurance (PPI). In a PPI scheme, contracting doctors and hospitals agree to negotiated prices (which they accept as payment in full) and utilisation controls. Insureds are given incentives to use these providers, and receive reduced insurance payments if they go to others. For example, such scheme might pay the fees in full for insureds who use preferred providers, but pay up to 80 per cent of those fees on behalf of insureds who use other providers, with the balance paid by the patient. The specific terms vary with employment group.

In 1983, Congress adopted the Prospective Payment System under which Medicare pays a fixed administered price for each inpatient case according to its Diagnosis-related Group (DRG). Payments are adjusted for area wage levels, and an extra allowance is paid to teaching hospitals. Originally, the payments were to be adjusted for increases in the prices hospitals pay. But hospitals reported record profits in 1984. In 1986, Congress decided to allow an increase of only one-half of one per cent for the following year even though inflation was higher. And less-than-inflation increases seem likely in the future. In 1984, Congress also froze the fees Medicare will pay physicians.

In its 1984 Budget, the Reagan administration proposed to limit tax-free employer contributions to employee health insurance. This was dropped in the administration's 1985 tax reform proposal, in the face of opposition from trade unions, the insurance industry, dentists and others whose economic interests would be disadvantaged. It is clear that there is widespread and deep resistance to the idea of limiting tax-free employer contributions to health insurance. But I believe the government will eventually be forced to do something to limit this source of revenue loss which is likely to exceed $50 billion in 1987 (Enthoven, 1986).

Employers have abandoned their hands-off stance and have become involved. For example, in 1982, Hewlett Packard Company in Palo Alto began to develop its own PPI scheme for those of its employees in the area not belonging to HMOs. In 1984 General Motors Corporation reached agreement with the United Auto Workers to add a PPI option. They subsequently announced that at the new Saturn plant, meant to be the 'factory of the future', employees would have only HMOs and PPI to choose from. Stanford Universtiy was offering its employees a cost-conscious choice among four HMOs and a traditional 'free choice' plan. In 1986, the University decided to replace the 'free choice' plan with PPI. Such developments led one Wall Street analyst to conclude, 'By 1990, the vast majority of the population will be in some such sort of health care delivery system, and fee-for-service medicine as we know it now will be dead' (Abramowitz, 1985). In addition, some employers are raising deductibles and co-insurance (the share of the bill the insured must pay). Many are examining the range of employee choices creating incentives for economic choice.

Physicians were so busy fighting 'socialised medicine' that they were 'hit on the blind side' by capitalism. The balance between supply and demand for physicians' services is tipping in favour of supply as cost-conscious demand meets the increasing supply. The condition of 'permanent excess demand' is being corrected. A generous supply of physicians is lubricating the transition in the delivery system to new organisational forms. The medical profession is now divided into many factions. The solidarity of the past is breaking up. More physicians than ever are willing to support non-traditional health care organisations. Professional autonomy is under attack from many sides including the economic, as employers, government, HMOs and insurers take advantage of advances in information technology to review physician performance in detail. In the 'guild free choice' era, there wasn't much an insurer could do about a doctor who, in its judgment, prescribed too many services, unless there was very serious and obvious abuse. Now, poor performers, including, for example, surgeons with high complication rates and re-admission rates, can be dropped from the preferred provider list.

Hospitals. The Medicare Prospective Payment System (PPS) and the growth of price-conscious selective buying of hospital services by CMPs mean that the cost-unconscious open-ended payer is disappearing. Hospitals are finding that they have no place to hide either the excess costs of inefficiency or excess overhead costs resulting from under-utilisation. (Unfortunately, it also means they have lost an easy source of payment for charity care.) A low occupancy rate used to be tolerable; it is becoming a disaster. And this is happening at the same time that inpatient use is declining. Hospital inpatient days declined nearly fifteen per cent from 1983 to 1985, and bed occupancy fell below 62 per cent in late 1985. So hospitals must improve efficiency and make deals with Competitive Medical Plans to attract patients. All this is easier said than done. It will require a drastic change in management culture. It used to be that the doctor who ordered every test known to man and kept patients in a long time, thereby running up the charges, was a preferred customer. In the world of PPS and CMP, he or she is becoming the enemy. Hospitals and doctors will have to team up to produce economical care to compete for contracts with CMPs.

HMO enrolment at the end of 1985 was 21 million, up 26 per cent from a year earlier, and double the 1981 level. While the per cent of the population served by HMOs is still small, at such growth rates this will change rapidly. As HMOs select economical providers and employ them efficiently, their margin of economic advantage over the traditional sector seems likely to widen. In 1986, about fifteen national HMO firms supplied the capital and management systems that enabled this pace of expansion to continue.

But the traditional sector is changing. Insurance companies had little to offer employers in the 'guild free choice' system. Employers found they were better off 'self-insuring'. PPI is a way for insurance companies to regain a marketable product and it is a way for traditional providers to compete with HMOs. The population size needed to realise economies of scale and for an adequate data base, is likely to exceed the size of all but the largest employers. So this is a market opportunity for insurance companies, and the largest companies have entered this field. In the mid-1980s, nobody yet really knew how to do PPI. The art of contracting between CMPs and hospitals was in a primitive state of development. I doubt that it is possible to select good quality economical doctors strictly by the numbers. But insurance companies have purchased or contracted with innovative software companies, and a great deal of creativity is being applied to the task.

There is no easy way to count the people covered under PPI arrangements because there is no legal definition or single agency (like the federal office of HMOs) to which insurance companies must report. But some indication of the potential is given by the experience of Blue Cross of California which started signing up

65

providers for its Prudent Buyer Plan in 1983 and three years later covered one million people. The four large investor-owned hospital companies purchased insurance companies and offered preferred provider insurance based on their own hospitals. By June 1985 they had enrolled a million people. One survey conservatively estimated total enrolment at nearly 6 million at the end of 1985 (Rice, de Lissoroy, Gabel and Ermann, 1985).

The conventional wisdom used to be that the transition of the U.S. health care economy to CMP was constrained by the ability of HMOs to grow some 10 to 12 per cent per year. On a base of less than 10 million, that could take a long time. By the mid-1980s, HMO membership was growing 20 to 35 per cent per year in key industrial states. PPI, which involves less investment and less organisation building, can grow explosively.

Cross-subsidies. By the mid-1980s, price competition was attacking two activities that were previously subsidised in part by cost-unconscious purchases of care: that is, charity or 'uncompensated' care of the uninsured and others unable to pay, and post-graduate medical education. (The Medicare PPS does include extra payments for teaching.) Hospitals burdened by high costs for these activities began to find their positions as economic competitors to be weakened. And they felt under growing pressure to cut them back.

WHERE THESE TRENDS ARE TAKING US:
TO MARKET COMPETITION

What will the health care economy look like in the year 2000? As my colleague Victor Fuchs puts it: 'Prediction is hazardous, especially when it is about the future.' So I offer projections of the implications of the mid-1980s trends, and not unconditional predictions. It is always possible that some other forces will emerge that will change the direction of the health care system. For example, if unregulated competition succeeds in destroying health insurance for enough people, there may be a more powerful political force for increased government action.

Government and employers, the main payers, will have brought the growth in their outlays for health care into line with the growth in their revenues. The simplest and most efficient way for them to do that will be by contributing fixed risk-adjusted *per capita* payments and offering consumers a choice of CMP, but leaving consumers cost-conscious in their choice. The share of GNP spent on health care will emerge from a balance of forces that includes an increasing average age, rising living standards, and new technology creating the possibility of new treatments on the expense-increasing side and competitive forces for efficiency on the expense-reducing side. Some new technology will be expense-reducing. The balance cannot be predicted. But I believe there will not be nearly such radical shifts in the share of GNP devoted to health care as occurred in the open-ended era.

Employers and government will have become much more sophisticated buyers of care. They will seek efficiency and equity for the populations they sponsor. The market system that will emerge will not be a 'free market' made up of health plans on one side and individual consumers on the other. Rather, it will be a market of 'managed competition' in which government, for the beneficiaries it sponsors, and employers, for the beneficiaries they sponsor, will contract with health plans to be offered to beneficiaries. These 'sponsors' will structure the offerings to their beneficiaries to make them intelligible and comparable, to control or compensate for risk selection, to assure continuity of coverage, to deter 'free riders' and generally to ameliorate the many serious imperfections that would inevitably plague a 'free market'.

Most *physicians* will find most of their practices through contracts with Competitive Medical Plans. Medical practice will be more closely controlled. Peer-reviewed clinical policies will be based on improved information about costs and outcomes. Medicine will be a little less art and a little more science. Physicians will be less priests and more technicians. Physicians will share power with managers.

Efficient Competitive Medical Plans now care for their patients with about one MD for 800 people. We are heading for a national supply of one active MD for 400 people. What does this mean for physicians' work and incomes? I do not think it will mean MDs driving taxis. But I think it will have an impact on incomes. CMPs paying doctors $50,000 per year will have a large price advantage over those paying $150,000. Physicians' incomes in the open-ended era were larger than needed to elicit an adequate supply of qualified persons. I believe market forces will bring physicians' incomes more into line with incomes of other similarly-trained professionals.

Many compensatory mechanisms will come into play. Doctors are the gatekeepers of the health care system. They can take back work they have delegated. We will see MDs running Intensive Care Units and replacing nurse practitioners. When a good general

67

internist can be hired for $50,000, it will not make much sense to substitute so many paramedicals for doctors. Lifestyles will change. When many physicians have husbands who are also doctors, 40 hours each will be able to support the family. Physicians will have more time for patients. They will need and have more time to read the medical literature. Quality-oriented CMPs will take continuing medical education more seriously.

A cost-conscious ethic will emerge. When people are given cost-conscious choices of health plan, many will choose less than the most costly standard of care. And their physicians' obligations will be to provide the standard of care their patients contracted for.

Hospitals will undergo many consolidations and mergers. If not acquired by CMPs, they will at least be working in close contractual relationship with them. Inpatient bed capacity will be shrinking from more than 4 beds per 1000 people towards the 2 beds per 1000 needed by efficient organisations. The market will force regional concentration of costly specialised services such as open-heart surgery where efficiency and improved outcomes can be realised. Hospitals will have shifted their focus from inpatient care to being the institutional base for comprehensive care systems.

The great majority of the population will receive its care through Competitive Medical Plans (HMOs and Preferred Provider Insurance). A variety in the systems and styles of care will persist, matching the variety in consumer and provider preferences. But there will be some narrowing in the range compared to what exists in the mid-1980s. HMOs and Preferred Provider Insurance will get to look more like each other in response to consumer demand. HMOs will find ways of accommodating members who want care from some outside doctors. And Preferred Provider Insurance plans will be based on increasingly cohesive organised medical groups whose contracts will include financial incentives for efficiency.

In 1985, Paul Ellwood predicted that 'within the next decade, delivery of health care in the United States will be dominated by as few as twenty national or regional medical care corporations, or 'Supermeds' . . . each responsible for the health of three to ten million people' (Ellwood and Paul, 1985). It is hard to know just where economies of scale run out. It seems clear that serving several hundred thousand enrollees confers economic advantages over smaller organisations. The largest health care organisation, Kaiser-Permanente, serving 5 million people, found it worthwhile to start several new branches in the mid-1980s. But there will continue to be strong regional HMOs serving several hundred thousand people each.

In sum, market forces will be working to solve some of our most serious problems and to give us a leaner more efficient health care economy. Consumer satisfaction will be getting a higher priority. Subscribers who are not satisfied with their care can switch to another plan at the next annual enrolment. In the mid-1980s, some health plans are using market research techniques to measure consumer needs, wants and satisfaction. Evening and weekend clinic hours are being scheduled to meet the needs of working people. Quality assurance teams interview patients to ascertain their perceptions about the quality of care received. Physicians who are uncaring or uncommunicative are identified and counselled.

In the HMOs and their competitors, physicians will accept major responsibility for controlling the quality and total cost of care. Strong effective peer review of the quality and economy of care will be in the physicians' interest. Under competition, physicians will voluntarily impose on themselves quality reviews and controls they would never dream of accepting if the government tried to impose them.

In the mid-1980s, the main unsolved problem in the American health care economy is that roughly 35 million people have no health insurance, public or private. If they cannot pay for care, they must rely on public providers of last resort such as county clinics and hospitals, or on charity care from private doctors and hospitals. (As noted earlier, competition is attacking the ability of private providers to subsidise such care. The taxpayer revolt is attacking the ability of public hospitals to provide it.) So the problem is not that they must go without any care at all; the problems are denial of access to timely care, financial hardship, and often a lower standard of care.

This problem is not technically insoluble, and it is not the inevitable consequences of a competitive market economy in health care. We could create public sector agencies to sponsor coverage for the uncovered. Demonstration projects have shown this is feasible. Through the tax system we subsidise health insurance for employed people. These tax subsidies are quite generous in the case of upper-income people because their coverages are extensive and they are in high tax brackets. We could restructure these subsidies to make them available to all Americans. The problem is in the willingness of American taxpayers and voters to pay more taxes to subsidise insurance for those now uninsured.

Our problem is not so much a lack of a shared belief that everyone ought to have access to a decent level of care. Our society recognises a public responsibility to assure such access. This is reflected in the Medicaid programme and local government provision of care to the

69

indigent. Nobody defends the gaps in coverage. The problem is that the translation of this belief into public policy has been uneven, inefficient and with gaps that seem arbitrary, the results of historical accidents. Somehow our society must resolve the conflict between the belief that everyone ought to have access to a decent level of care and our national preference for decentralised private markets and local solutions to social problems.

ACKNOWLEDGEMENTS

The author gratefully acknowledges the financial support of the Henry J. Kaiser Family Foundation and the assistance of Pauline Burton, Laura Gardner, Gregory Vistnes and Nancy Wilson in the preparation of this chapter.

REFERENCES

Abramowitz, K. (1985) *The future of health care delivery in America*. Bernstein Research, New York.

Ellwood, P.M. and Paul, B. (1985) 'Here comes the Supermeds'. *InterStudy*, Excelsior, Minnesota.

—— Anderson, N.N., Billings, J.E., Carlson, R.J., Hoagberg, E.J. and McClure, W. (1971) 'Health Maintenance Strategy'. *Medical Care, 9*, 291–8.

Enthoven, A.C. (1978) 'Consumer Choice Health Plan'. *New England Journal of Medicine, 298*, 650–8 and 709–20.

—— (1986) 'Health Tax Policy Mismatch'. *Health Affairs, 4*, 4, 5–14.

Feldstein, M.S. (1970) 'The Rising Price of Physicians' Services'. *Review of Economics and Statistics, 52*, 121–33.

Fleming, S. (1973) *Structured competition within the private sector*. Unpublished memorandums within the Department of Health Education and Welfare, Washington, DC.

Havighurst, C. (1978) 'Professional restraints on innovation in health care financing'. *Duke Law Journal*, 1978, 304–88.

Luft, H.S. (1978) 'How do Health-Maintenance Organizations achieve their "savings" '. *New England Journal of Medicine, 298*, 1336–43.

Rice, T., de Lissovoy, G., Gabel, J. and Ermann, D. (1985) 'The state of PPOs: a national survey'. *Health Affairs, 4*, 4, 25–39.

Sapolsky, H.M., Altman, D., Greene, R. and Moore, J.D. (1981) 'Corporate attitudes toward health care costs'. *Millbank Memorial Fund Quarterly/Health and Society, 59*, 561–85.

Weller, C.D. (1984) ' "Free choice" as a restraint of trade in American health care delivery and insurance'. *Iowa Law Review, 69*, 1351–92.

Wennberg, J.E. and Gittelsohn, A. (1973) 'Small area variations in health care delivery'. *Science, 182*, 1102–8.

6

Economic Issues in the New Zealand Health System

Michael Cooper

After nearly fifty years of comparative stability (in contrast to the Australian health care system which has undergone seven structural changes since 1975), the New Zealand health care system is now going through a period of intense questioning and re-examination of both its objectives and underlying assumptions. The last serious attempt at comprehensive reform came to grief in 1974 when a White Paper was vociferously condemned as a copy of the British NHS (*Health Service for NZ*, 1974). Predominantly state funded since 1938 (85 cents in the health dollar comes from taxation[1]), the system is now suffering from a widespread resistance to both the level of taxation and, more particularly, the manner in which it is raised. Very high rates of inflation, with the exception of 1979, in excess of 15 per cent every year between 1976 and 1982, have driven nominal incomes up through steeply progressive tax rates. During this period, the mounting tax burden has been increasingly borne by persons liable to PAYE, with the result that this section of the public now tends to regard taxation as rather more akin to confiscation than to the public price of public goods and services, and consequently are becoming increasingly unwillingly to pay in taxation for the services that they continue to demand as patients.

High inflation plus little or no indexing of the income tax thresholds yielded, until comparatively recently, substantial and annual sums to the public coffers (through fiscal drag) together with mounting budget deficits, which supported rapidly growing public expenditure. In 1984, inflation dropped to 3.5 per cent (but returned to 13.4 per cent in 1985) and with it fiscal drag and a renewed determination to reduce a budget deficit which had reached nearly $3,000 million or just under 9 per cent of gross domestic product (GDP). In addition, the new government pledged to cut personal income tax (maximum marginal rates are to fall from 66 per cent to 48 per cent on incomes of $38,000 plus from this October) and to introduce a form of VAT (GST). Against this background, it is perhaps not surprising that total health spending, having grown steadily from 2.9 per cent of GDP before the war to 6.8 per cent by 1981, has since declined to 5.6 per cent. Indeed, since 1981, state expenditure on health has declined both as a percentage of GDP (from 5.8 per cent to 4.9 per cent) and as a percentage of government expenditure (from 12.07 per cent to 9.86 per cent), largely giving way to increased transfer payments and expenditures on social welfare. Whereas total health expenditure in real *per capita* terms (namely State, Accident Compensation Corporation and private expenditure on health adjusted for movements in the CPI) grew between 1974–78 by 13.29 per cent and between 1978–82 by 12.76 per cent, since 1982 it has actually declined by 12.97 per cent.

Pressures on tax funding have in turn led, of necessity, to a vigorous questioning of the health care system, its organisation, aims and achievements. Faced with real cuts in expenditures, the efficiency with which money is used has been called into question, with Hospital Boards feeling that the same health care provision for less expenditure has been often confused with less for less. Indeed, lowering the percentage of GDP devoted to health has been in danger of almost becoming an objective in itself. In this climate of opinion, it has been hard to keep the real question, namely, whether the last dollar spent on health yields more or less satisfaction than that forgone, to the forefront of the public mind. One by-product of financial stringency has been a growing emphasis, at least in debate, on the causes of mortality and morbidity rather than on their treatment. Although we still lack a fully integrated model of the variables which interrelate to determine the health status of a given population at risk, a systematic pulling together of available epidemiological and econometric work clearly suggests that the socio-economic variables have been traditionally grossly understated (Cooper, 1981). In the future, increasing emphasis is likely to be put upon influencing life-style decisions as to smoking, alcohol consumption, exercise and nutrition. These and other variables such as pollution, housing, unemployment, education and income distribution are the outcomes of past individual and collective choice and as such are potentially amenable to change. These choices, however, are often complex, involving trade-offs between competing ends. Prolonging life is no one's sole objective and may conflict with the quality of life as perceived by the individual in question. Cars, for example, are seen as essential to our social and commercial interaction but they also kill 600 to 700 New Zealanders every year. Further, smoking gives pleasure to a third of our citizens but it also kills some 3,600 a year (15 per cent of all deaths). Clearly, although the rules of healthy living may be well known, they do not appear to be widely held as being particularly inviting. There is both a limit to the quantum of resources that we are prepared to divert to prolonging life, and to the number of 'sacrifices' of pleasure that we are prepared to make to that same end, although recently both smoking and alcohol consumption appear to be in decline (Alcohol Liquor Advisory Council, 1985; Hay, 1984).

Although rising real expenditures on health care do not necessarily lead to increased life expectancy, they do affect our quality of life and, in particular, the level of care provided to those in various dependency states (e.g. dying, being born, handicapped or chronically ill), which forms more than 60 per cent of health service activity. The quality of these services is undoubtedly threatened by falling resources. Further, somewhat paradoxically, although when health expenditures were increasing improvements in life expectancy tapered away to virtually zero, as health expenditures have first plateaued and then declined, significant improvements have again been recorded. These gains are, no doubt, in part a reflection of life-style changes and of the rapid improvement in the life chances of the Maori population (8.8 per cent of the total population of 3.3 million). The gap in life expectancy between non-Maoris and Maoris fell by 63 per cent for males and 58 per cent for females over the period 1950–82. A significant difference still remains of 68.29 years to 70.66 years for males and of 72.43 to 78.81 years for females, but to an extent this continues to reflect life-style differences (e.g. 58.6 per cent of Maori women smoke compared with 27.6 per cent for 'others').

In common with the United Kingdom, the founding fathers of our health care system tended to assume that, given current medical knowledge, the health needs of the population were quantifiable and finite. Although in any one year some needs may go unmet, the goal of meeting all need was, in theory at least, considered potentially attainable. The major problem in a socialised system was thought to be persuading the population as a whole to surrender sufficient purchasing power to the state to meet the full needs of the sick. In reality, however, there exists no unambiguous and finite quantum of medically assessed need. The more resources the state makes available, the greater the professionally assessed need is likely to be. That is, need is thought to be continuously reassessed in the light of scientific progress and available resources. Within a largely zero-priced or heavily subsidised system such as New Zealand's, a large continuum of latent demand always exists, held in check by access costs and professional assessment of need. Both of these checks are themselves influenced by the severest rationing device of all, the sheer availability or otherwise of labour and resources. Such thinking was, at least in part, responsible for the introduction in 1981 of a population based funding formula as a means of distributing Vote: Health amongst the competing claims of New Zealand's then 29 Hospital Boards.

Until comparatively recently 'Vote: Health' was distributed very largely on the basis of individual Board estimates of their financial requirements to maintain current services plus their bids for new services. The Department of Health would aggregate such claims and compare them with Vote: Health, adjusting individual Board aspirations to available funds as proved necessary. Under this system, service provision became very uneven over the country and any inequalities largely self-perpetuating. Further, given the annual real growth in funding, zero budgeting was not attempted and overall objectives seldom stated. Capital works, once given central permission, became public borrowings with both debt servicing and eventual repayment a charge on the Central Consolidated Fund. Indeed, once opened, any new building attracted a commissioning grant which was henceforth incorporated into the base of the Board's recurring allocation. Such a system, not surprisingly, resulted in a system strongly oriented towards institutionally based health care. With the reversal in funding trends came the desire to find a more robust indication of need than a simple aggregation of Boards' bids for resources. An indicator of *relative need* was required rather than individual Board's views of *absolute need*. The answer was thought to lie in a population based funding formula broadly similar in type to the English RAWP system.

Local assessment of need, it was argued, simply reflected the resources already on the ground whereas population numbers would reflect a more objective and independent assessment of relative need. The problem, however, has been that the implied redistribution of resources between Boards adjudged on the basis of the model to be overfunded to those underfunded, has had to be attempted during a period of overall decline. Overfunded Boards have faced real cuts in resources rather than, as would have been the case during a period of growth, small or zero increments. In the event, actual redistribution has had to be modest causing mounting frustration at the slowness of adjustment amongst potential gainers but doing little to dampen the cries of anguish from the rest. It is in the nature of such models that although the basic assumptions upon which they are based may be wholly plausible they are none the less of necessity largely arbitrary in nature, and in danger of sometimes leading to highly precise but potentially misleading conclusions. Once created, such models appear to have a life of their own. However arbitrary the underlying assumptions may have been thought initially, once in place they tend to be regarded with a degree of unhealthy respect. This model is based upon an estimation of a Board's predicted share of total national bed days (for other than psychiatric and maternity beds, this is determined by population share weighted by age and sex, and adjusted for variations in standardised mortality ratios). The model includes further adjustments for cross-boundary flows (at national average bed-day costs), private and voluntary beds (discounted to 75 per cent), bed days for those over 65 years old (discounted to 62 per cent), regional or national specialties and teaching hospitals. Its major flaw lies in the fact that New Zealand's 3.3 million population is divided amongst 26 Hospital Boards and 3 Area Health Boards with individual populations ranging from 2,100 to 800,000 people. These Boards have grossly different responsibilities, dissimilar provisions of private facilities, significant variations in case-mix, ethnic composition, cross-boundary flows, teaching beds and so on. To make matters worse, the over- and underfunded regions (South and North respectively) are neatly divided by a line running across the country just north of Wellington adding yet further spice to already well developed North–South rivalries. Indeed, the drift of population north has meant that overfunded boards such as Otago (11 per cent overfunded) have found themselves moving no nearer to equity despite suffering repeated cuts in funding. The Otago Board has argued vigorously that although it does not oppose funding models in general, it is seriously disadvantaged by a number of the features of the existing one. The model, for example, assumes need and population to be linearly related, and that there are no economies associated with either large-scale health provision or high population densities. Otago, like other Boards, is reimbursed at national averaged bed day costs (i.e. $240) for its net cross boundary flows but 23 per cent of its admissions, mostly complex and relatively expensive cases, are from outside its borders. Over 65 per cent of its cardio-thoracic surgery, for example, is performed upon imported patients at a cost of $552 a day and this discrepancy alone accounts for $1.6 million of its asserted $8 million plus overfunding. Further, the Board feels that in compensating for the presence of a teaching hospital, no allowance is made for the impact of such a hospital on both case-mix and the sheer volume of services generated by the presence of a large range of specialists and equipment (i.e. additional supply creating both extra need and demand). In contrast, Otago gains from the somewhat illogical inclusion in the model of SMRs (standardised mortality ratios) which weight excess deaths despite the fact that it is not death which costs the Board money but life. Many handicaps and chronic diseases are expensive to treat and relieve but these costs are not reflected in higher mortality ratios (e.g. mental illness and handicap, diabetes, MS, etc). Further, underfunded Boards argue that cross-boundary flows should be adjusted at marginal and not average costs. The question remains, however, as to whether taking 100 people away from a Board of 100,000 and placing them in a Board of 800,000 is likely to have the same impact, one positive and the other negative, on their respective costs of health care provision, and whether a population based formula can be made to work in a system in which 50 per cent of the Boards have populations of under 50,000. Inefficiencies are inevitable when real cuts have to be made rather than achieving equity through differential growth rates. Cuts are made where they can be rather than where ideally they should be. Even if demand and need do tend to reflect supply, the transitional strains of downward adjustment are bound to be severe.

The disenchantment with need as an independent variable is also apparent in the renewed interest being shown in medical labour planning. Three or four years ago, the government of the day and the profession were united in their desire to cut medical school intakes but for diametrically opposed reasons. The state believed that every additional doctor qualifying would generate additional demands upon the service, whereas the profession believed that the more doctors in the field the less work there would be for each, thereby causing downward pressure on medical incomes. In the event, medical school intakes were cut with the aim of reducing the annual output from 320 to 250, but the current government, rather in the manner of the Grand Old Duke of York, has recently increased the figure to 270. Labour planning has been seriously hampered by the fragmentation of the exercise into a series of investigations each embracing a single profession, and by a lack of overall agreed health care policy objectives. Unless the overall objectives are clear, it is impossible to do more than speculate as to each profession's proper contribution towards their attainment. Variations in the ratios of medical personnel to population, for example, are such as to suggest that the tasks performed by health workers are far from uniform across the country. In 1983, the number of doctors per 100,000 varied from 37 in the Maniototo and 53 in Dannevirke, to 206 in Wellington and 311 in Otago, and the number of general practitioners from 1 to 2,700 in Invercargill to 1 in 1,700 in Whangarei (their consultation rates varied from 2.5 to 4.7). The number of persons per physiotherapist varied from 3,100 in one Board area to 11,100 in another. In 1984, there were 38,000 people per ophthalmologist in south North island and 83,000 in south South Island; 20,700 per psychiatrist in south South Island and 52,000 in central North Island; and 23,100 per internist in south North Island and 70,800 in south South Island. The labour power and cost implications of standardising to the lower, higher or middle of these ranges are clearly dramatically different. Further, retention of trained staff in the face of higher overseas rewards and and the seemingly inbuilt urge of all New Zealand young to travel has caused mounting difficulties. A third of New Zealand's medical graduates have emigrated since 1960 and retention rates amongst nurses and physiotherapists are similarly poor. The average working life of a registered nurse is 17.5 years and 6–10 years after registration 72 per cent of occupational therapists and 55 per cent of physiotherapists are no longer professionally active.

One of the major obstacles to the formulation of clear national policy has been the fact that, despite the state providing 85 per cent of total health spending, the actual provision of health care is split into a complex pattern involving the state (Hospital Boards, new Area Health Boards, and District Health Officers) and subsidised private and voluntary sectors. Despite the growing emphasis given to community care during debates on priorities, hospitals continue to dominate total health expenditures, having increased from a 60 per cent share in 1960/1 to a 74 per cent share in 1984/5. Hospital services are divided between 170 public (24,485 beds) and 174 private hospitals (6,514 beds or 21 per cent of the total) (Department of Health, 1985). Although beds have been decreasing (from 102 beds per 10,000 in 1980 to 94 in 1985), the decrease has been entirely in the public area (Department of Health, 1980 and 1985). Private bed numbers, however, have recently been made subject to a measure of public scrutiny and control, largely in recognition of the adverse affect their rising numbers have on Hospital Boards through the operation of the Allocation Formula. Public hospital beds decreased by 10 per cent in the ten years ending 1985 but patient admissions rose by 22 per cent, outpatients almost doubled and day patients trebled. These trends were not achieved without placing considerable stress on staff with the inevitable sporadic outbursts of unrest particularly amongst junior doctors.

The gatekeepers to the whole system, the 2,284 general practitioners (or 1,841 full time equivalents), operate in a subsidised fee per item of service 'private market'. Relations between them and the state have also been far from cordial in recent months due largely to disputes as to the adequacy and appropriateness of the 'general medical services' benefit (GMS). The profession maintains that this subsidy or benefit, which for adult consultations has remained at $1.25 since 1972, falls to the patient and not to the profession, whereas the state has been reluctant to increase the amount largely on the grounds that to do so would in practice benefit the patient very little. The dispute came to a head last year when the government increased the benefit for child consultations from $4.75 to $9.50 on the condition that current consultation fees (including subsidy) were held in check so that the gap between benefit and fee was in effect limited to about $2.00. This 'control' was resisted by all but some 500 doctors and so an attempt was made to restrict the increased benefit to the patients of this more amenable group. This was subsequently successfully challenged in the courts on the grounds that children attending other doctors could not legally be denied the new benefit. In the event, the state chose not to amend the legislation in the light of the court's ruling but to increase the benefit to $10.50 for all child consultations on the 'understanding' that it would be passed on to the patient in full. No threat of statutory sanctions against defaulters, however, now exists. The long running dispute as to who benefits from the GMS, doctor or patient, has resulted in only one change to the adult benefit (from $0.75 to $1.25 in 1972) being introduced since the scheme's introduction in 1941. The original intention was that the subsidy would normally meet the fee in full, but since that time it has dropped in value from a sum equal to 7.5 per cent of the average weekly wage to only 0.39 per cent. Indeed, to have maintained its real value since 1941 it would now have to be $13.15. In fact, regardless of whether the formal incidence of the subsidy is on the patient (as it is in a very few medical practices where the doctor declines to bulk bill the state) or on the doctor, the actual incidence is likely to be shared, with the doctor receiving somewhat more, and the patient paying rather less, then would have been the case in the absence of the subsidy. This system of paying general practitioners, who have no contractual obligations to the state, is unlikely to last more than two or three years. The state is unlikely to put further public money into primary care until agreement is reached on a new system, probably along the lines of a dual capitation (to compensate for practice expenses of approximately 50 per cent of gross income) plus a fee per item of service (subsidised only in the case of especially targeted groups).

The falling real value of subsidies, the introduction of prescription charges (in 1985 at $1 per item with a similar range of exemptions to those found in the UK), and a growing waiting list for elective surgery in public hospitals, has contributed to a rapidly rising volume of private health insurance cover. From being virtually unknown in the 1960s, private insurance now covers at least 35 per cent of the population. In dollar terms, however, it remains relatively modest at less than 2 per cent of total health spending and contributes only 35 per cent of private hospital surgery costs. No doubt the trend in coverage was accelerated by a combination of a wage freeze and increasingly penal income tax rates which made it easier and more advantageous for employers to include benefits of this kind than to grant wage increases but, surprisingly, employer contributions towards premiums remain little more than 15 per cent.

The original intention of the 1938 Act was to subsidise private hospital beds so that the benefit to the patient was 'the same amount as would have been payable in respect of that treatment if it had been afforded by a Hospital Board' (Social Security Act, 1938). Whether such a position ever existed in practice remains in some doubt but today subsidies account for, at best, some 37 per cent of geriatric and medical, and 19 per cent of surgical expenditures. The notion that subsidies should go some way towards recompensing patients for their tax contributions towards a public system that they have chosen not to use, still persists. Subsidies to the private and voluntary hospitals are many and complex having been built up over the years in a piecemeal rather than in a planned and co-ordinated manner. The daily patient benefit is important ($26.50 for surgical and $25.50 for geriatric patients) as is the assistance given towards costs on income related grounds, such as the Geriatric Hospital Special Subsidy Scheme for those admitted to a private hospital when no suitable public accommodation is available. Payments are also made by the Department of Social Welfare which is prepared to contribute towards the cost of up to 28 days hospitalisation per year for a patient normally cared for at home (as relief for the home carers). In practice, the private sector provides 50 per cent of all geriatric beds, treats 30 per cent of all accident cases requiring hospital treatment and performs 25 per cent of all surgical operations. Surprisingly, despite the rapidly rising insured population, the percentage of operations performed in private hospitals actually fell slightly between 1978 and 1981, from 25 per cent to 22 per cent, before recovering last year to their 1978 level.

Accident victims requiring general practitioner or private hospital treatment have their fees paid by the Accident Compensation Corporation. The ACC, introduced in 1972 on the advice of the Woodhouse Report (1967), is responsible for the single biggest source of distortion in the current health care delivery system. Designed to provide compensation, rehabilitation and prevention from personal injury from any cause and funded from an earners' scheme, a motor licence surcharge and, for the non-earner or visitor not otherwise covered, from the Consolidated Fund, the Scheme has produced an elite set of highly favoured 'patients'. There is the growing unease as to why patients should be treated so radically differently simply on the basis of whether they have walked into a virus or a bus. Further, the habit of the ACC of paying for private hospital treatment on the grounds that this avoids prolonged earnings-related compensation whilst victims, absent from work, await public hospital admission, is now also being seriously challenged. Total real ACC expenditure on health care has increased 185 per cent since 1975 (over 80 per cent since 1980). The main impact has been in orthopaedic surgery where private hospitals now undertake 30 per cent of all procedures. In 1982, the ACC circulated a list of surgical procedures, mostly orthopaedic, for which it would 'accept immediate responsibility for private hospital admission and reasonable cost associated with the treatment given' (ACC, 1982). For other procedures, inability to obtain treatment in a public hospital within three months was to be treated as sufficient justification for a private hospital admission. In practice, this has had the effect of attracting specialists into private practice (on part tenths from the public hospitals) thereby lengthening the waiting lists further and sometimes causing difficulties in finding sufficient beds to train, in particular, orthopaedic surgeons. Prior to the ACC, there were few private physiotherapists but by 1985, 50 per cent of practising physios were in the private sector many earning 90 per cent of their incomes from the ACC. There are now more than 90 vacancies in the public sector, more in fact than the total 1986 output from the training schools, and public services are having to be cut back still further. The stress caused by shortages is in turn causing further retention problems. Apart from superior financial rewards, private sector work involves no shift work, few domiciliary visits and for the most part healthy patients whose injuries are frequently self-resolving.

The basis on which medical charges are to be determined is not specified in the ACC legislation but in practice has related to a device known as the 'annotation line' (i.e. practitioners having to 'annotate' aspects of a case which they consider would justify a higher fee than 'normal'). Initially, the annotation line was widely seen as generous and, indeed, is thought to have had an inflationary effect on fees charged by general practitioners to all patients. Now the ACC fee is intended to meet only '95 per cent of fees customarily charged' (ACC, 1985). The ACC itself is expressing concern that doctors are seeing patients more than is strictly necessary and that cases with an element of doubt are being too readily classified as accidents. Since 1981, for example, ACC claims have increased 22.5 per cent but related doctor services by 40 per cent. Probably over 20 per cent of general practitioner incomes now originate from this source. Similarly, physiotherapists' services increased 63 per cent and the associated costs by 241 per cent (Morel, 1985).

Rumours are now rife that the ACC is about to introduce a series of changes including a much sterner interpretation of what constitutes an accident (although the costs of case policing could prove formidable); leaving victims to make significant part-payment towards their treatment costs; and re-directing some 15,000 patients to the public wards (or more accurately, to the public waiting lists). The probabilities are that the whole process of discriminating between sickness and accident may be softened by providing ongoing limited support on a common basis for all those disabled from whatever cause. Carers might be subsidised whether the care is provided at home or in an institution. The lack of compensation for sickness 'injury', however, would remain.

THE FUTURE

The health problems of New Zealand are largely those that would be anticipated in a highly developed nation operating a predominantly socialised health care delivery system. Tax revenue is becoming harder to find at just the time when the population is ageing. Those aged over 65 years will increase some 40 per cent in the next twenty years and, more importantly in terms of resources, those over 80 will almost double. The evidence is that for those over 65 the major illnesses requiring care and treatment increase almost exponentially with age, and the normal period of dependency prior to death extends significantly. This group already consumes four times *per capita* the health resources of the rest of the population. Health expenditures should be growing at least 1.7 per cent per annum in real terms merely to maintain the same *per capita* level of service to a growing and aging population.

Until recently the rise of private insurance cover and the advent of the ACC were changing the basic nature of the health service almost by default and certainly without debate or declared intent. The problems of the system, however, are now being investigated by a positive deluge of committees of inquiry. Public Committees are now actively investigating health benefits, the ACC, medical labour planning and the education of nurses. A Royal Commission to examine the whole basis of social policy has recently been announced. The Department of Health has just completed its first formal corporate plan, which should form a solid basis for the formulation of future national health policy. A revamped Board of Health, with eleven standing committees, has been formed to advise the Minister on medium and long term planning which will hopefully lead to a clearer statement of the main health objectives and the most cost-effective means of achieving them. In the meantime, three Area Health Authorities have been created (Northland, Nelson and Wanganui) under recent enabling legislation, involving the merging of Hospital Boards and District Health Offices (outposts of the Department of Health) and incorporating the private and voluntary sectors directly into planning through the establishment of multidisciplinary service development groups. Further, a rationalisation project has just been launched in the south South Island involving six Hospital Boards, which will hopefully lead to the eventual formation of the fourth Area Health Board.

Despite all this activity, the next twenty-five years are unlikely to bring any dramatic structural or funding changes. The 26 remaining Hospital Boards are likely to evolve slowly by a process of voluntary amalgamation into a maximum of 10 Area Health Boards. This process will in itself make the Allocation Formula considerably easier to operate as variations between these enlarged Boards with respect to population size, case mix and service responsibilities will be drastically reduced. General practitioners will probably be persuaded, largely by economic necessity, into accepting a more formal relationship with the state. In return, state benefits for consultations will be returned to a level where they cover at least 75 per cent of total doctor charges. The ACC will increasingly direct accident victims into the public hospital system and reimburse doctors at approximately 75 per cent of their 'normal' patient consultation charges. Smoking in public places and drinking to excess will become more universally socially unacceptable. The great unknown, of course, is the future trend in New Zealand's *per capita* income which will in turn determine the future availability of tax revenue. It is this above all else which will determine the balance between the public and private sectors. Certainly the period of financial uncertainty since 1980 has concentrated the collective health mind wonderfully, recalling the observation, commonly attributed to a great New Zealander of the past, Lord Rutherford, 'that in the absence of any money there is little option but to sit down and think'.

ACKNOWLEDGEMENT

My thanks to Mrs M.L. Berkeley and Mrs N.J. Devlin for assistance with the research upon which much of this chapter is based.

NOTE

1. All references are to New Zealand dollars.

REFERENCES

Accident Compensation Corporation (1982) *Medical Bulletin no. 19*, May.
———— (1985) *Medical Bulletin no. 45*, August.
Alcohol Liquor Advisory Council (1985) *New Zealand Alcohol Consumption Statistics*, Wellington, NZ.
Cooper, M.H. (1981) 'The economics of health'. In J.G. Richards (ed.) *Primary health care and the community*, Longmans Paul, Wellington, NZ.
Department of Health (1980) *Hospital management data*. National Health Statistics Centre, NZ.
———— (1985) *Hospital management data*. National Health Statistics Centre, NZ.
Hay, D.R. (1984) 'Smoking and health'. *Report no. 40*, National Heart Foundation of NZ.
Health Service for New Zealand (1974) Government White Paper,

Wellington, NZ.
Morel, V.M. (1985) 'Who pays for health?' Paper presented to the NZ Institute of Health Administrators, November.
Social Security Act (1938) Section 93, p. 87.
Woodhouse Report (1967) *Report of the Royal Commission of Inquiry on Compensation for Personal Injury*. Wellington, NZ.

7

Health Economics in Japan: Prospects for the Future

Shiro Fujino

BACKGROUND FOR COST CONTAINMENT AND THE BASIC PROBLEMS

Between the 1960s and the beginning of the 1970s, Japan enjoyed the highest rates of prosperity in which top priority had been given to material growth in shaping political objectives, while health and welfare promoting policy had been given lower priority. However, having attained considerable economic growth with materials in reserve, peoples idea of life changed from a quantitative one to a qualitative one, and consequently the national policy began to put greater emphasis on welfare.

In 1973, ironically when Japan suffered the first oil crisis, the government declared it the first welfare year and put into practice the free health care cost programme for the aged. Back in 1961, a compulsory health insurance system had been introduced which accelerated the demand for health care services even though the charges were partially borne by the people. It had been argued that the supply of health care (especially of doctors) could not catch up with the rapid growth in the demand for health care, and that the doctors' influence upon market performance was fairly major. As a result a series of new medical schools were authorised from the 1970s. In the first half of the 1970s, welfare services were expanded and it was decided that the new technology should be principally applied immediately in the insurance service, regardless of its high cost, and as mentioned above, an increase in the number of doctors was also decided upon. Since 1973 when the brakes were suddenly applied to economic growth, the expansion of public welfare services has become one of the major factors in the rapid increase of a 'red ink' bond resulting in financial deficit in the 1980s. In the

1980s the ageing of the total population has become a major social problem. Health care costs for those over 65 are relatively higher than those of other age groups and, with the maturing of pension programmes the burden on the people will increase sharply in the future. Moreover, a comprehensive health care system for the aged will not be established in spite of the government policy.

In thinking of the future of health economics in Japan, it can be safely said that there are four issues: the demand for and supply of health care services, the government financial deficit and the ageing of the total population. Since the ageing of the total population can't be controlled by a policy, it is considered a given factor. (Therefore, this will be a key factor in future health economics.) As for the financial deficit, the government will take measures to decrease public services and to keep a balance between benefit and burden in terms of health care cost containment. In the next place, the supply of health care could be controlled to some extent by policy-makers. For instance, there are annually about 8,000 newly qualified doctors at present and they plan to reduce this by 10 per cent, which is to be put into practice without fail. It is impossible to control technical progress, but it is possible to control the introduction of new health care technology into the health insurance service programmes by policy. The Medical Law was revised in 1985 in order to modify the health care system with a view to cost containment. Lastly, the demand for health care services can be controlled to a certain extent by raising co-sharing of health insurance. Indeed, in 1983 the Insurance Law for the aged was introduced, according to which a fixed but small amount of the partial burden was imposed on persons over 70 and those aged between 65 and 69 who are bedridden, namely ¥400 per month for outpatients and ¥300 per day (2 months) for inpatients. Consequently, the demand (the rate of care-received) was actually controlled, but this only continued to be effective for about a year. It showed that the psychological effect of being obliged to pay even a small portion of what had until then been free, was greater than the effect of the real burden amount itself. In 1985 the Health Insurance Law was revised and as from October of the same year 10 per cent of co-sharing was imposed upon the insured (about 35 per cent of total population) who had been covered 100 per cent till then. The relative success of this practice will be revealed with the passage of time. It appears to be effective in terms of control at present.

EXTREME ACCELERATION OF AGEING AND THE DEMANDS FOR HEALTH CARE SERVICES

The ageing of the total population is the result of the reduction of birth rate and the increase in life expectancy. The latter might be one of the indexes of quantitative improvement of health. However, it does not necessarily mean its qualitative improvement. Actually, the proportion of those who are sick has steadily increased in conjunction with the above fact. Let us look more closely at the relation between the life expectancy, aging and the proportion of sick people to healthy.

The average life expectancy of men in 1960 was 65.3 years and of women 70.2 years and since then it has continued to increase reaching 74.5 and 80.2 years respectively in 1984 (Ministry of Health and Welfare, *Life Tables*). Incidentally after the Second World War life expectancy was 50 and 54 years. This shows that there has been a remarkable increase in life expectancy since the war, and more importantly, it also shows the difference between the rate of increase of youth from age 0 to 14 and the rate of increase of the aged over 65. In 1984 the number of those aged over 65 was 12.63 million while in 1960 it had been 5.3 million. This shows an increase of 2.4 times (Statistics Bureau). On the other hand, the number of those under 14 in 1984 was 26.32 million while in 1960 it was 28.07 million, representing a decrease. This rapid change in the structure of population in only 25 years has made the incidence of disease change drastically. There is a sharp increase in adult diseases such as cerebral apoplexy, cancer and heart disease. (In 1985 the death rate from cancer was 156, from heart disease 117.3 and from cerebral apoplexy 112.2 per 100,000 (Ministry of Health and Welfare, *News Report*)). In Japan as the number of aged has increased, the probability of occurrence of chronic invalids has also increased as a result of the increase in life expectancy.

In order to confirm the above, let us examine the changes in the number of people with diseases (Ministry of Health and Welfare, *National Health Survey*). The rate of people with disease (per 1,000, hereafter the rate of disease) shows an increase of 290 per cent between 1960 and 1984, from 46.9 to 137.3. Even though the rate of disease is influenced by influenza epidemics and economic fluctuation, a clear up-trend is evident over this 25-year period. The fact that the rate of disease increases by 2.9 times while the number of those over 65 increases by 2.4 times suggests that the increase in the rate of disease might be explained by the increase in the number of the aged. This is easily confirmed by examining the rate of disease according to age group. The categories consist of ten-year groups except the categories of those under 14 and over 75. From 1962 to 1984, the curve of the rate of disease of the age group 15–24 remains bottom, and the curves of other groups move upward with increase of age. And those of the age groups 65–74 and over 75 have been quite high (the figures for 1960 and 1961 are not available). The rates of disease of age group 15–24 in 1962 and 1984 are 27.2 and 35.1 respectively. On the other hand, the rate in the ages 65–74 increases from 145.6 to 424.1 and that of over 75 increases from 123.2 to 556.8. In these 23 years the difference in the rates of disease between the young and the aged has increased by from 4–5 times to 12–16 times. These facts make clear that the increase in the number of the aged is the principal factor which gives birth to the increase in the rate of disease. (In connection with this, disease of organs of circulation shows a higher rate than other diseases.) A clear up-trend can be confirmed when a diagram of correlation between the number of the aged over 65 and the rate of disease (especially of the aged over 65) is drawn. While the rate of disease is not necessarily the index of the quality of health, the quantitative increase in health, with the increase of average life expectancy, has been accompanied by a decline in quality of health in Japan.

What is more important is that the trend in the rate of disease indicates the trend of potential demand for health care services. The Institute of Population Problems of the Ministry of Health and Welfare estimates that in the year 2000 the total population will reach 128 million, of which the number of over 65s will be 15.6 per cent of the total. In other words, the number of those aged over 65 will amount to 20 million (Ministry of Health and Welfare, 1981). As mentioned above, there is a positive correlation between the rate of disease and the number of the aged. Since the saturation point in the rate of disease has not yet been reached, a steady increase in the rate in the coming 15 years can be foreseen. This means that the potential demand will continue to increase. Naturally, not all the potential demand is actualised. The actual demand in Japan can be observed, to some extent, through the rate of care received (per 100,000 of population) which is published by the Ministry of Health and Welfare (*Patients Survey*). This rate shows an increase of 1.5 times from 4,805 to 7,427 between 1960 and 1984. In 1960 the rate was 4,317 for those in the group of age 65–74 and 4,168 for over 75s. In 1984 it has risen to 15,064 in the group aged 65–69 and 21,517 in the over 70s. In these 25 years, the rate of care received by the aged has increased by 4–5 times, although it is not possible to compare directly the data of 1960 and 1984 due to different categories of ages being used. Though the rate of care received does not show so much change as the rate of disease, the trend is the same in the case of the aged. The change in the rate of care received by the aged is mostly due to the change in the rate of disease of the aged. Here, it is clearly seen that there exist causal chains showing that the increase in the number of the aged in these 25 years produced the increase of the rate of disease and that it produced the increase in the rate of care received. It suggests that it will not be an easy matter to control the demand for health care, which will be a key measure in controlling health care cost in Japan, due to the rapid expansion in the numbers of the aged in the coming 15 years.

TREND OF HEALTH CARE COSTS

The trend of health care cost will be examined here (Ministry of Health and Welfare, *National health care costs*). Until 1975 the rate of growth of health care costs had been high and there were several years in which it reached up to and over 20 per cent per annum. After 1975 (when the rate was 20.4 per cent), the rate steadily decreased, and in 1984 the rate of growth was 3.8 per cent. The health care cost per head grew from ¥4,400 in 1960 to ¥125,500 in 1984. As the matching of the growth curve to these figures is good, it seems that it was getting to saturation point at the beginning of 1980s. However, the saturation is mainly the result of controlling the increase in the cost of manpower and hospitals since 1975, especially in the beginning of the 1980s, aside from the argument of whether it is the result of the law of decreasing returns in the health care sector (Koizumi, 1979). As for the standard prices of medicine in health insurance services, they decreased by about 50 per cent during these five years and since medicine forms a high percentage of the national health care costs in Japan, these price reductions have helped to control health care cost to some extent. Since the latter half of the 1970s the government has taken a number of measures to control costs, the most effective of which was control of the cost of manpower and hospitals.

The health care costs of age groups are quite different. These data are available from 1977 (dental costs and costs for pharmacy are excluded). In 1977, the cost per head was ¥67,600. While the cost per head of the group under 14 was ¥27,700, that of the group over

65 was ¥219,000, which is 3.2 times as much as the average and 8 times that of the under 14 group. In 1984, the average cost per head was ¥109,700. Though the cost per head of the under 14s increased to ¥40,300, that of those over 65 grew to ¥394,300 during these seven years. The cost per head of the aged was ten times as much as that of the group aged under 14 in 1984 and, moreover, the total cost of the over 65s (10 per cent of total population) is 35.7 per cent of the total health care costs. The cost in cases of hospitalisation of the aged over 65 is 41.9 per cent of the total for the aged. The ratio is higher than those of other age groups. One of the main reasons is that the aged stay longer in hospital. The average length of stay in general beds was 39.3 days in 1984 and many of the aged stay far longer than that.

It can be said that the control of the growth of health care costs focusing on the matter of payment to doctors and hospitals shows good results so far, but control of the trend of increasing costs of the aged does not necessarily show good results.

CONCLUSION

In the years until 2000, the population of over 65s is sure to increase by 7 million and the rate of disease is also sure to grow. Potential demand to expand health care further, a part of which will certainly be actualised, will also occur. Above all, the cost per head for the aged will without doubt be quite high. From all of this we expect that the main issue of health economics in the near future will be the problem of the health care costs for the aged.

The issue of health care for the aged is not simply that of cost. The reason why the aged stay longer in hospital is that there is not enough space for three generations of a family to live together and the young are not in favour of taking care of aged parents because of the development of the nuclear family. Furthermore, there are not enough nursing homes available. At present, the total number of nursing homes have a capacity of only two hundred thousand. Due to the shortage of nursing home places, the aged tend to occupy general beds in hospitals for a long time.

The Ministry of Health and Welfare has been promoting in-house care for the aged as a means of curbing costs. However, this seems unlikely to be effective because of reasons outlined above. Meanwhile, the Ministry is hammering out a plan for setting up 'intermediary facilities', a new concept which aims to shorten the long stays of the aged in hospital, curbing the increasing cost for the aged. It will, however, take time for this plan to be realised.

For the time being, the only means by which the government could curb the health care costs for the aged would be a change of the forms of out-of-pocket money contributed by the aged from the small flat-rate to a fixed rate of the total costs, holding the rate to around 10 per cent. If this impossible, health care costs will continue to increase at a higher rate than the GNP until 2000. Though the aim of the government is to keep it on a level with the rate of growth of GNP, it will be difficult to do so, because they have already made every effort to curb costs. Towards the year 2000 other factors such as the introduction of new technology, including new medicine, development of self-care, and improvement of health care delivery systems will have an influence on our health, but it must be stressed that in Japan the most important issue in the health care sector in the future will be the rapid increase of the aged within a very short period.

REFERENCES

Koizumi, A. (1979) *Cost-benefit analysis of medical care in the welfare-oriented society*. Proceedings of the 2nd meeting of the WMA follow-up committee on development and allocation of medical resources, Japan Medical Association.

Ministry of Health and Welfare, *Abridged life tables 1960–84*, Statistics and Information Department, Tokyo.

—— *11th life tables* to *15th life tables*, Statistics and Information Department, Tokyo.

—— *National health care costs 1960–84*, Statistics and Information Department, Tokyo.

—— *National health survey 1960–84*, Statistics and Information Department, Tokyo.

—— (1981) *New estimates of future population*, Institute of Population Problems, Tokyo.

—— *News report on 1986 vital statistics of population*, Statistics and Information Department, Tokyo.

—— *Patients survey 1960–84*, Statistics and Information Department, Tokyo.

Statistics Bureau of Management and Coordination Agency, *Population census of Japan*, 1960–80.

—— *Population estimates as of 1 October 1961–84*.

8

Health Economics and the World Health Organization

Brian Abel-Smith

The World Health Organization has been slow to make use of the skills of health economists. In the early days of cost-benefit analysis when some health economists arrogantly assumed that all that mattered was the economic benefits of health programmes — lost earnings as against the direct costs of health intervention — the subject was not surprisingly given a cool reception in Geneva. Moreover some excessive claims were made for conclusions built up on the assumption that if hard epidemiological data were not available it was acceptable to make guesses. It is because of some unfortunate experiences of this kind that economists were slow in gaining acceptance in the health field. But over the years acceptance has grown. There are currently eight on the staff of the World Health Organization in Geneva most of them working on specialised problems such as tropical diseases, the economics of water programmes, drug supplies, family planning and the planning of the campaign against river blindness (onchocerciasis) in the Volta valley which is likely to be the second major success story following the world abolition of smallpox. There are also some health economists in regional offices.

From December 1983, financial planning at the macro level has moved to the centre of the stage. It is simply because this is a relatively new development that the rest of this chapter is devoted to this programme. This is not to imply that economic support for particular health programmes is any less important. But such work has been long established and the more sophisticated forms it can take are reported elsewhere in this volume.

Macro economic work has a long history in the organisation but for many years it was regarded simply as research. A pilot study to compare health expenditure and sources of finance in six countries was published in 1963 (Abel-Smith, 1963) and followed by a wider study in 1967 (Abel-Smith, 1967). Further studies were made in particular countries and the whole field was reviewed by a study group which met in November 1977 and recommended that countries should be urged to undertake periodic surveys of financing and resource allocation in their health sectors as part of their health planning processes (WHO, 1978). This was followed by a series of workshops, consultation meetings and seminars (both regional and international) at which the uses of studies of financing and planning resources were promoted. The findings were brought together in two manuals published in 1983 (Griffiths and Mills, 1982; Mach and Abel-Smith, 1983). A special issue of *World Health Statistics Quarterly* reviewed progress at the end of 1984 (World Health Statistics Quarterly, 1984). Up to this point the actual work done in particular countries rarely extended beyond the collection and analysis of past data. Often data were incomplete covering only the public sector or excluding some or all health-related activities. Moreover such studies were, in most cases, special *ad hoc* exercises rather than a continuing activity built into the planning process. Rarely were they used as the basis for forward projections of expenditure in order to work out the long term cost of meeting planned objectives and to find out how the proposed health programmes could be paid for.

The strategy of Health for All 2000 published in 1981 called upon Ministers of Health to establish a financial master plan for the use of all financial resources after examining all possible sources of finance (WHO, 1981). Some twenty countries were encouraged to cost their plans as part of what were called 'country resource utilisation reviews' but in many cases the data were hurriedly put together and were difficult to relate to existing expenditures. Making cost projections was also emphasised as part of the promotion of programme budgeting. Where countries did attempt to cost their plans, they often lacked credibility simply because the sources of finance were unspecified or left as a future gap, often a very large one, for foreign donors to fill.

The new thrust to promote financially realistic plans for health for all came for two main reasons. First it became clear during the first attempt to monitor progress towards health for all how few developing countries could even attempt an estimate of what proportion of gross national product they were spending on health services and that a high proportion of the estimates which were provided were unreliable or seriously incomplete. But the second and most compelling reason was the World Economic Crisis. Health for All was launched in 1977 — still a time of economic optimism: only in the case of the countries of sub-Saharan Africa was there any doubt among international agencies about the prospect of a continuing rise in the living standards of developing countries. Moreover there was a hidden assumption that much more financial support for the health programmes of the developing countries could be attracted from richer countries if the case were well presented.

It therefore came as a shock to discover that between 1981 and 1983, average gross domestic product fell by about 9.5 per cent in Latin America and by 11 per cent in sub-Sahara Africa and that there were also falls in living standards in the least developed countries of Asia. During the same period low growth in Western Europe and North America had led to a massive increase in unemployment.

The fall in living standards exposed the extent to which developing countries had fallen into debt. Devaluation and high interest rates made debt charges a formidable prior charge on government budgets amounting to up to a third or a half of export earnings. While some countries fought valiantly to maintain the level of their health budgets or even increase them, austerity policies drove the majority of developing countries into cutting expenditure on the health sector. In addition balance of payments deficits forced many countries to cut imports of medicines and medical equipment.

At the same time, the industralised market economies were saddled with the problem of maintaining millions of unemployed, most of them young. This created a crisis in social security financing: more people needed maintenance, while there were less people at work paying taxes and contributions to support them. Thus in these countries also containing the cost of health care became an overriding objective of policy. In these circumstances, budgets to help poor countries develop their health programmes were competing with extra heavy demands on public expenditure at home. As a result there was virtually no increase in external aid to the health sector.

Some African countries, faced with the formidable consequence of drought on top of all their other problems and the virtual disruption of their rural health services began to lose faith that Health for All was possible — or at least by the year 2000. One suggested that the year 2100 might be more appropriate. There was a real danger that Health for All would remain a dream unless countries were prepared to face up to the problem of limited resources and plan within totals of what further resources could realistically be expected to be made available, both internally and internationally.

Thus a new programme was launched within WHO under the somewhat uninformative title of 'Economic Strategies to Support the Strategy for Health for All'. The programme was made a main item for discussion at the Executive Board in January 1986 and at the World Health Assembly in May 1986 and will have a follow up in the form of a technical discussion at the 1987 World Health Assembly. The essential messages which the Organization is seeking to promote are the following. First, countries need to know what is being spent on the whole of the health sector, public and private, and how it is financed. Second, the extra cost of Health for All plans should be calculated as uncosted plans amount to no more than window shopping. Third, that countries should investigate every possible source of finance for paying for the plan. Fourth, where necessary, plans should be revised downwards to fit the resources which could realistically be expected to be made available and every step taken to make better use of existing resources and to find the most cost-effective way of achieving particular health objectives.

All this may seem so obvious that it hardly needs stating, let alone promoting as a world programme. But remarkably few countries have in fact a costed health plan and by no means all that have one have faced up to the question of how it is going to be paid for. An unduly optimistic plan contains a number of dangers. First, highly qualified staff may be trained in large numbers only to find later on that they cannot all earn their living either in the public sector or in the private sector. This wastes both training costs and human resources. Secondly, political pressures may lead to paid jobs being found for surplus doctors and the money found by cutting both training for and staff complements at lower levels of qualification. Thirdly, costly buildings, particularly hospitals, may be built but when they are complete money may not be available to equip, staff and supply them at an adequate level. Or, if the money is found, this may be at the expense of developments of higher priority such as extensions in primary health care. Fourthly, staff may be trained and given jobs but grossly insufficient supplies of drugs, petrol and equipment to use their skills effectively. There are many examples of each of these planning errors in developing countries today. The aim must be to avoid repeating these mistakes.

Faced with all the uncertainties, some countries are reluctant to attempt to plan for more than a few years ahead. But a longer term plan, up to the year 2000 is needed for three reasons. First, the number of highly trained staff which can be financed in the long run should determine the educational programme for the next five years.

95

Secondly, the number of hospital beds whose running costs can be found in the year 2000 must determine the number of beds built over the next five years. Thirdly, any major redeployment of resources which may be thought too painful or politically contentious if carried out over a short period may be more acceptable if phased over ten years or more, during which vacancies caused by retirements can be left unfilled and younger staff retrained for other tasks.

The most creative part of the planning task is the search for new or further sources of finance. The essential problem is that it is unlikely that developing countries will be able to find much more money out of taxation unless the economic fortunes of the Third World change radically for the better or the health sector is given much higher priority. This is unlikely to happen in view of the demands of other sectors of development. Moreover additional taxes which are regressive can be counterproductive to health development. Nor are there any signs that there will be a massive increase in foreign aid to the health sector. Even if donors can be found to help with capital developments, this still leaves the running costs to be found and these are the major costs in the long run.

The possibilities for further funds differ according to the way in which health services are organised and the traditions of the different countries. In some there may be opportunities for stimulating further support for non-profit organisations or creating new systems of local informal insurance or revolving funds (e.g. for drugs). A further possibility is to increase the yield of existing charges or introduce new charges particularly geared to help secure a more efficient use of current resources. Some developing countries charge far below cost for the use of private rooms in government hospitals. In some countries modest charges for drugs may be the only practicable way to discourage excessive prescribing. Other charges may be geared to discourage patients going direct to the hospital, bypassing on the way their local health centre. Substantial charges levied at the hospital for non-emergency cases with exemptions for cases referred from the health centre may help to secure a more economical use of the health care system. If services are only well developed in urban areas and some rural areas have no services at all within reasonable access, it seems only equitable that charges levied at urban services should be used to help finance extensions of services to the rural areas provided ways can be found of exempting the urban poor.

A further possibility which is attracting increased interest is the development of new schemes or further schemes of compulsory health insurance. This option has been discredited among many public health experts in view of the unfortunate effects caused by health insurance in so many countries of Latin American. At its worst health insurance can be extremely socially divisive: it can promote sophisticated curative services heavily weighted towards expensive hospital care for the regularly employed (mainly the urban population) and provide such generous remuneration for doctors and others that it becomes extremely difficult for Ministers of Health to recruit staff to work in rural areas or provide the critical preventive services which should be of highest priority in both urban and rural areas. What does not, however, follow is that it is impossible to devise schemes which do not have these adverse effects.

The essential case for compulsory insurance is that if ways can be found for those in the modern sector and their employees to pay the full cost of the services they use, tax money can be released to extend rural services to those uncovered or inadequately covered at present. But what is crucial is to avoid creating financial incentives which make it harder to recruit staff for rural services. One way of avoiding this is to confine the right to work for health insurance to staff who have completed a substantial period of rural service or to make the extent of insurance practice allowed depend upon the duration of the rural service which has been completed.

Over the past decade, new schemes of health insurance have been started in Korea, the Philippines, Thailand and Indonesia though not all these schemes meet the above criteria. There are currently new plans for health insurance in Syria and Zimbabwe. Not surprisingly, these schemes take many different forms. Some build on earlier precedents while others have been specially devised to meet the requirements of the particular country. The solutions which countries choose to adopt will inevitably depend on what is politically acceptable. The question of charging for health services is politically contentious in developing countries as it is in countries already more developed. A scheme which works well in one country such as the sale of health cards to the rural population which give rights to free health care many never get off the ground in another. A country with strong rural co-operatives may be able to build an informal health insurance scheme as one of the functions of co-operatives. Much depends on what is administratively feasible. Schemes of workmen's compensation are commonly found in developing countries. This may be an administrative base upon which compulsory health insurance could be developed.

WHO is not only encouraging developing countries to look at all these alternatives but providing consultant support in analysing all possible options for consideration by countries which have requested this form of help. Similar assistance is being given by the World Bank and the Asian Development Bank. Consultant help is also being given with the costing of health plans. It is expected that demands of this kind will grow as a result of the prominence currently being given to the importance of financial planning.

Why do countries need help of this kind? The planning units of the Ministries of Health of developing countries are generally staffed by personnel who have had postgraduate courses in public health — many of them in France, Britain and the United States. And many of the curricula for local public health courses were modelled on courses in these countries. Their grave weakness was the failure to include relevant teaching, and in many cases any teaching at all, in health economics. Thus planning departments often lack both the competence and confidence to handle the financial aspects of planning. On the other hand finance departments have developed to service Ministries in their short term functions of preparing annual budgets and then controlling them and accounting for them once appropriations have been obtained. Persons with skills in financial planning are seldom found anywhere within the staffs of Ministries of Health.

What has therefore come to light is a major deficiency in training. And new short courses have been developed to provide Ministry staffs and others with the opportunity to build up knowledge and competence in this area. Moreover it is now recognised that for staff entering the field of health planning a good grounding in the macro aspects of health economics and an awareness of the capabilities of economic appraisal will be essential. The World Health Organization has been discussing this with the World Federation of Public Health Associations. Schools which accept the importance of making this addition to their curricula will need to recruit staff or arrange for the training of existing staff to teach in this area. Thus there is a further need for courses — in this case to train the trainers.

Health economics has largely developed in the industrialised countries — particularly in the United Kingdom and the United States. There are extremely few health economists so far in developing countries. The focus of teaching and research in the United States has inevitably been on the working of private markets and competitive insurers subject to a minimum of regulation. Health economists from the United Kingdom where the working of the National Health Service and all the consequential problems of trying to allocate resources so as to secure both efficiency and equity have long been studied and are therefore in a strong position to help develop health economics in developing countries where the public service model of providing health care has been widely adopted. Moreover Europe contains a wide variety of different schemes of regulated national health insurance from which lessons can be learnt about their problems and the ways which have been found to try and overcome them. All this experience can be of considerable value to developing countries considering options for the future financing of their health services.

Beneath all the rhetoric, the Health for All programme is essentially the application of health economics to health policy making. The problem is how a society can maximise health out of limited resources and secure the equitable distribution of health benefits. It became recognised during the 1970s that certain health interventions were known to be extremely cost-effective though they were not being made available to the whole population. These were listed as the eight essential elements of primary health care and packaged together as primary health care programmes — the key to achieving Health for All by the Year 2000. The emphasis on community participation was also based on cost-effective principles as in democratic societies you cannot even take the horse to water, let alone force the horse to drink.

It is only in the last few years that the World Health Organization has recognised that health economists can assist in helping put these principles into practice. The earlier failure to accept help was partly due to some health economists claiming much greater competence and understanding of the health field than was in fact the case. Health economists will only be accepted in the long run in the WHO, Health Ministries and health insurance agencies if they have the humility to accept that they still have much to learn.

REFERENCES

Abel-Smith, B. (1963) 'Paying for health services'. *WHO Public Health Papers no. 17*, Geneva.
——— (1967) 'An international study of health expenditure'. *WHO, Public Health Papers no. 32*, Geneva.
Griffiths, A. and Mills, M. (1982) *Money for health*. Sandoz Institute for Health and Socio-Economic Studies, Geneva.
Mach, E.P. and Abel-Smith, B. (1983) *Planning the finances of the health sector*. WHO, Geneva.
WHO (1978) *Technical Report Series, no. 625*.

────── (1981) *Global strategy for health for all by the year 2000.* Geneva.
World Health Statistics Quarterly, 37, 4, 1984.

9

A European Health Policy for the 1980s and 1990s

Herbert Zöllner

During the period of colonial independence and post-war reconstruction every country was proud of its particular health care system and equated its growth with progress. It was only at the beginning of the last decade that the suspicion was heard that continued health care investments at the present magnitudes might not bring the desired health yield and, indeed, might not be able to be financed. This situation, which eventually reached crisis dimensions in several developing countries, led the World Health Organization to take a critical look at its overall policy and to propagate the worldwide goal of health for all by the year 2000 (HFA2000).

While the overall situation in Europe was less serious, marginal productivity appeared to be declining rapidly. The member states of the WHO European Region (which includes northern, western, central, southern and eastern Europe as popularly defined plus, for the last few years, Israel) therefore decided to analyse the particular health problems of rich industrialised countries and to search for innovative measures to secure health in the future. The results of this scientific work, which had been carried out with the help of several hundreds of experts from 25 disciplines and had involved numerous discussions with leading politicians in member countries, was a memorable event: the 32 countries decided to adopt a common health policy in Europe, the so-called Regional HFA2000 Strategy. It was stressed that this was not a supranational policy but a policy that countries would make their own and adapt to their particular circumstances.

Cynics who had predicted that implementation would stop at the declaratory level were wrong. At the moment of writing, about two years after the adoption of this policy, more than half of the European countries are taking a critical look at their own national and subnational health policies and are reformulating them in the light of the European policy and its 38 specific health targets. It augurs well that these countries represent all parts of Europe, and that interest is growing in other countries. Each country reports every three years on progress in implementation and health development.

The aim of the European policy is the same as the worldwide aim, namely to achieve a level of health that would permit each citizen to participate satisfactorily in economic and social life. In Europe, however, more emphasis is put on health as a major dimension of quality of life as well as on popular participation, and thus the reduction of inequalities in health risk exposure, health service use and health status, is a major principle. This pertains not only to health-related differences between countries, such as, for example, between France and Turkey, but also the inequalities in health between social groups inside a country. Single-parent families, the disabled, long-term unemployed, unskilled workers and other socially weak groups should also be enabled to participate in economic and social life.

The European health policy consists of four main lines of approach. The first line is the promotion of health-relevant lifestyles. The most important health problems in Europe relate to the ways in which its people live, whether or not they are addicted to tobacco and other substances, how they eat, drink, exercise, drive and so on. The policy calls upon countries to put considerably more emphasis on health promotion and development. That this is feasible can be seen in the reduction in smoking achieved in a number of countries, such as the United Kingdom, Norway, the United States and Finland, where heart attacks and strokes have been reduced similarly.

The second line of approach is an active policy of environmental health protection, including a better management and perception of health risks. Europe is fast running out of pollutable reservoirs, and an increased number of chemical substances pose major health threats. The recent nuclear reactor accident in Chernobyl and its radiation load on Europe illustrate the need for internationally concerted action.

The third line of approach is a shift of the balance of health care in favour of primary care in the community, at home and at work, with less reliance on closed institutions. This is not a call against inpatient care and medical care in general but for substitution wherever possible without loss of quality, by outpatient care, by care delivered by other professional providers and, indeed, by self-care, family-care and support by self-help groups.

The fourth and last line of approach is the mobilisation and management of the above-mentioned HFA2000 strategies by an appropriate mix of incentives, long-term health planning and scenario building, technology assessment, policy analysis, information, interdisciplinary research, inter-sector collaboration, popular participation and discussion, manpower planning and resource allocation. It is in this policy and management support that health economics has an important role to play.

THREE FACES OF HEALTH ECONOMICS

Health economics deals with the economic aspects of health activities. While this definition appears to be straightforward, 'economics' itself can be thought of as a topic, a discipline and an everyday practice or behaviour.

Economics as a topic is the study of certain aspects of the economy; that is, the production, trade, consumption and distribution of goods and services. The scope of health economics encompasses such activities occurring within the health sector, for example, the organisation and financing of health services, the functioning of health centres and hospitals, and the ways in which health and health services are produced and distributed in the population. Work in this area is difficult; it requires a good understanding of health care institutions and epidemiological relationships in practice.

As a discipline, economics is characterised not so much by the subject matter but by the method of analysis. In this sense, economics is a social science which analyses the costs and consequences of a wide range of human endeavour and seeks to explain, forecast and sometimes prescribe the allocation of resources. The cornerstone of the discipline of economics is the concept of choice: choices are essential because resources (people, time, facilities, equipment, knowledge) can be used in various ways and are scarce in relation to all wants and needs. For example, economists assess the effectiveness and equity of health strategies and measures in reaching their overall aim of better health, and the efficiency with which health resources are utilised. Economists working in the heatlh area require special proficiency in economic theory and policy in order to distinguish the areas where standard economic principles apply without modification and the areas where they may need rethinking and retooling.

In their daily life, people often demonstrate economic behaviour. One is constantly confronted with choices involving trade-offs between the advantages and disadvantages of particular actions. Everybody therefore practices economics some of the time, uses some general economic concepts and information and may even seek the advice of a professional economist. However, it is by no means easy to become an intelligent consumer and lay practitioner of economics: cost cutting and parsimony, common examples of the popular notion of economics, are not necessarily wise economic measures. In the health field, there are additional difficulties. Health care, often painful, brings little pleasure in itself, except in the case of jogging and body-care and certain other preventive actions. On the other hand, the consumer is often ill-placed to judge the likely health benefit and places choice into the physician's hands, who in turn may be less certain about outcome than he or she claims and may be influenced by other considerations and incentives as well. Furthermore, is there another sector of the economy with a comparable lack of economic information?

In the following, an attempt will be made to sketch the future development of health economics in Europe.

The topic of health economics

If one compares the subject areas in the health field that are systematically covered by economists to the European health policy agenda, then it becomes evident that there are quite big gaps in health economics work.

Health economics will need to widen its frame of investigation beyond conventional health institutions and services if it wishes to remain policy relevant. One may therefore predict that health economics increasingly will take up topics related to the promotion and production of health and the management of health risks. As an example, the Regional Office has recently initiated a study on the economics of tobacco, alcohol and drug addiction. In the area of prevention, health economics will increasingly focus on the other sectors of the economy and the economic implications of various mixes of incentives and guidelines for health and the sectors concerned. Also tackled will be the more difficult area of community-wide interventions into several risk factors simultaneously and their implications for efficiency and equity.

There remains ample scope for health services economics as well.

One does not have to look at the United States of America to see that there are changing patterns of medical practice, supply, organisation and finance. Three questions in particular will demand attention: should health care financing be more closely related to type of patient served and, if so, would it be useful to have a price per type of patient episode inside and outside hospitals? Should we introduce more competition within the health sector and, if so, how could this be done within the public sector? Should we give more resources and thereby economic power to primary health care and, if so, which sectors should be suffering?

It is well known that richer countries spend proportionately more on health services, but this is not necessarily true in the rich 'European league'. Economists will want to take a close look at whether spending little more than 6 per cent of GDP in one country represents under-funding (cutting services and quality?) and around 10 per cent in another country over-spending (gross inefficiency and provider oligopolies?) National health accounts are notoriously inadequate, in spite of heroic attempts at standardisation, notably by OECD. A compromise will have to be found between the Standard National Accounts (and therefore production-oriented accounts) and health policy purposes, which deal with health in functional (consumption-oriented) terms.

Health economics as a discipline

Health economics suffers from the inadequacies of some areas of economic theory. For example, immunisations and other preventive health services do not fit the standard image of services that are consumed the same instant they are produced. The concepts of time and need, never fully and adequately dealt with in general economics, pose special problems in the health field. It is here that progress is desired: the European health policy is a long-term policy; given its nature, it is also couched in the normative language of 'prerequisites', 'needs', 'recommendations' and 'targets'. When it comes to health policy inside countries, however, success will depend on the ability to link yearly negotiations about budgets or fee schedules (to give examples of short-term preoccupations) with the longer-term cost-effectiveness and cost-benefit implications of health strategy options.

Regarding the promotion of economic information, the Regional Office pursues two lines of activity. The first is to try to identify innovative approaches regarding the measurement of economic aspects of performance (effort, efficiency, cost-effectiveness and aspects of equity and effectiveness) of health care within a territory, for a given group of population and inside a health care institution. The second is to learn how countries do in fact monitor the allocation of resources to their stated priorities (such as care of the elderly, non-communicable diseases, primary health care). In addition, WHO supports studies of health care financing and programme budgeting in some of the less privileged member states in Europe.

The Office has also supported the recent issue of *World Health Statistics Quarterly* (December 1985) that is devoted to economic evaluation in the health field. The methodology is by now quite established but some of the 'finer' points will be strengthened by European economists in the near future. Firstly, there is now more economic analysis and measurement of health status. Since there now exists some work in QALYS and utility measurement, why not also help operationalise WHO's HFA definition of 'participation in economic and social life'? We may well see an economic epidemiology of health. At present, we do not know whether the health services are in the same predicament as Alice in Wonderland who had to run in order to stand still (meaning that economic growth creates so many additional health problems that it is a defensive victory for health services to maintain health at the earlier levels) or whether health services become less and less relevant instruments of health policy à la McKeown.

Second, more attention is being paid to systems boundaries that are implied by different policy questions, e.g. some of the methodological dissent disappears if one asks 'what are intervention options to bring people at risk or ill closer to those in normal health, and what are the consequences (excess consumption, deficit production, welfare losses, all seen relative to health peers)?' The most important part in policy analysis and advice is to get the issues right. And it seems to be quite biased when questions are addressed to prevention that are not also asked of curative services, such as whether the action 'pays for itself'. Economists will continue to address the 'societal level' but will more often refer to the viewpoints of different groups. Even regarding the societal level, they will take a more balanced view that health services and goods are both a cost and a benefit to the economy. More generally, strategic options will be stimulated for both partial and general equilibrium points of view. Important in this connection is also economic information about whole episodes across providers and institutions, not only instances of care.

Third, ideal-type options and readily available options will be more clearly distinguished. There will be less 'normative ideology', which often compares one's ideal with the other's 'dirty reality', such as many advocates of either market competition or state planning are using. And there will be more focus on choosing the appropriate mix of options (even if 'second best'), and in designing incentives and strategies to achieve the transition from the present system (for example, hospital 'savings'). Also, especially in the area of technology and pharmaceutical assessment, there will be more analyses of the consequences of pushing the margin beyond the originally foreseen and tested areas of application.

Fourth is the shift in analysis from spending to resource allocation. There are few studies on the cost to consumers of care, and yet time costs are considerably larger for middling patients than the few marks (substitute your favourite currency) of 'cost sharing'. Many cost-effectiveness studies still use average spending per bed-day when examining different inpatient strategies. The emerging consensus that 'indirect costs' are not important to decision-making will be overturned, as it appears to be a result of myopia when working on magic formulas about how to break down a health services budget into smaller and smaller units.

Fifth, with regard to financing in 'rich Europe', there will be more work on the incentives of different financing systems and their effects on the behaviour of physicians, nurses, patients and hospital administrators, to mention a few actors. Of special interest are also the implications of spending ('cost') control/containment for quality, access (geographical, between social groups) and health outcomes. The Regional Office is working on hospital, dental and primary medical care. Incentives will become the most important health organisation topic in all parts of Europe.

Sixth, there will be better economic analysis of health research. There will be less copying of research approaches from the United States, where the many small pilot projects require a special 'microscope type' research. In order that researchers may learn from each other, next year the Regional Office is launching an HFA2000 research plan, and setting up networks of researchers. Randomised controlled trials require careful planning and preparation. The longer the chain of causes and events, the less clear the research hypothesis (for example, some experts appear to argue in favour of randomising for both understood and not-understood factors), the less economic aspects are taken into account, the more

107

the trial is likely to fail and to yield misleading conclusions. Randomised trials should be compared to other research options, such as systems analysis. This is not a cry against randomised controlled trials, but a hope that trial designs will be subject to economic analysis as well, and that research questions will target in on the areas of uncertainty that could make a difference in the decision at hand. Economic analysis will increasingly be involved not only before and during the clinical trial but also afterwards when the transition has to be made from the research 'laboratory' to the real world and its resource limitations. Also, there will be more scope for experimentation in the economic aspects of health activities themselves (especially in organisation, management and financing), in line with the conclusions of a WHO meeting on budgetary incentives for the appropriate technology of health.

Finally, economists will be less pretentious: they do not have all the answers to the questions they pose; it is not enough to have the master model of costs and benefits. Economists will collaborate more often with political scientists, sociologists, epidemiologists . . . even if it will not always be possible to agree on a joint methodology and may mean that the same real-world phenomena are illuminated from different angles. Furthermore, there will be more health economists, that is professional economists specialising in the health sector, as the importance of the health sector in the economy would appear to warrant. The reasons for this are, now that the health sector share of the economy has grown relatively large, some of the newly developed economics tools or principles can be more readily applied to the health sector, and the centres of power are less firmly occupied by physicians and other health professionals.

It will be less often the case, therefore, that lawyers, physicians, statisticians, engineers and others having no proper training or experience in economics will be forced to fill the vacuum left by economists. On the other hand, the same lawyers etc. will make excellent allies in interdisciplinary work, as has already been demonstrated in some countries. The Regional Office has supported informally or helped to establish a number of professional health economist associations in Scandinavia, Spain, Portugal, the Federal Republic of Germany, and Mediterranean countries, and is arranging a workshop with Eastern European economists in 1987.

It should not be forgotten in this connection that Europe also has an important task *vis-à-vis* the developing countries, which have an appalling shortage of economists in the health field. The Regional Office will therefore embark on establishing a network of Europeans who are qualified and wish to work in this area.

While health economists in different countries use similar concepts and methods, they differ in the subjects they tackle: economists in Britain tend to take up issues regarding cost-effectiveness, in Sweden regarding the impact of ill health on the economy, in the Federal Republic of Germany regarding the cost of social security, in Mediterranean countries regarding gaps in incomes and in access, in the Federal Republic of Germany regarding the cost of social security, in Mediterranean countries regarding gaps in incomes and in access, in the Soviet Union regarding the appropriate levels of norms and standards, and in the Netherlands regarding regionalisation. Most health economists are health care economists, that is, they deal with the management, financing and use of health care services. They will be more concerned in future with the production of health by means of changes in the social and physical environment, an area of increasing policy interest.

The present economic climate poses similar questions regarding basic health and social policy in the context of different countries: how far can the costs of health and social care be rolled back to the individual families? Which types of health care should be safeguarded even in times of cutback? Should the health sector increasingly become an outlet for excess labour and high-technology equipment? Will better health promote economic growth even in a situation of significant unemployment?

In order to answer these and the policy questions mentioned earlier, economists will join with other disciplines. To be inter-disciplinary one needs (i) a sufficient number of health economists who are knowledgeable in economics and understand the major issues in health; (ii) a representative number of health care providers, managers and administrators who are able to look beyond their narrow disciplinary and institutional boundaries, include in decision-making an economic way of thinking, and act as informed consumers of health economics; and (iii) collaboration throughout the policy formulation process, thus avoiding economists being called in too late, when the decision has already been made or when the only mandate is to cut costs somehow.

Health economics as a behaviour

The changing climate in the economy of the health sector

When health care resources were plentiful, physicians, nurses and other health care providers did not know much about the economics of health. They could help their clients with any procedures they thought beneficial, however small, while at the same time making a decent income and having good social standing. When governments attempted to control costs, physicians found ingenious ways to ignore or sidestep these controls. Since the late 1970s, however, economic constraints have been felt increasingly in the physicians' workshops: cost control is succeeding in many countries, the number of health care providers is becoming more abundant relative to population, and (net) physician incomes are increasing less rapidly than average national wage rates. Nurses in several countries have taken up economic arguments, in order to help justify their professional roles in the care of the elderly and the chronically ill, and in defence of their income claims.

Similarly, hospital managers had little incentive to economise, since any 'reasonable' costs they incurred were reimbursed in practice, regardless of whether the hospital happened to be paid by patient-day or global budget. It is now less fashionable to consider deficits as the normal state of affairs, there are more attempts to compare performance across hospitals, and managers have begun to bargain harder with external suppliers. Managers are also beginning to introduce modern methods of cost accounting and to contemplate giving economic incentives to health care providers.

Similarly, until recently, administrators working in national, regional and local health departments did not have to defend the allocation of society's resources in the same 'hard-nosed' economic way as administrators in other sectors of the economy; instead they could hide behind the façade erected by the care providers, namely that health, like human life, has no price, and that therefore almost any budget increase could be justified by appeal to this moral imperative. This has also changed: increasingly health administrators find themselves in competition with other sectors of the economy as regards investments and in conflict with local communities when it comes to cuts in services. Administrators, therefore, make ample reference to costs, savings, efficiency and other economic aspects.

Society will be unwilling to spend more on health care without getting commensurate value for money.

New skills in health economics

The changing climate in the economy of the health sector demands that health care providers, managers and administrators learn to understand the relationship between the economy of their units and the economy of the health sector and, ultimately, the national economy. They also have to ask of themselves — and, where professional skills are required, ask of economists — the relevant economic questions, and to introduce these questions into the processes of decision-making at appropriate times and in an appropriate manner. In brief, they have to go beyond their narrow clinical, institutional and bureaucratic boundaries, learn to use an economic way of thinking in decision-making and become informed consumers of economics.

Health care providers

The primary economic skill of health care providers should be the recognition and acceptance of cost-effective strategies, whether health-promoting, preventive, therapeutic, nursing or rehabilitative. They should also understand the difference between a 'technical' approach (that is, continue to doctor or nurse a patient as long as there is any benefit to be gained regardless of cost) and an 'economic' approach (continue only if the additional benefit justifies the additional cost). A third economic skill should be the providers' recognition that they are agents on behalf of their patients collectively as well as individually: health care delivery is a process that is not only technically determined but also behavioural and discretionary. In a similar way, general practitioners, public health physicians and community nurses should be aware of their important agency role in interfacing with other sectors (e.g. traffic safety, nutrition) that have an impact on the health of their clients and people in general. A fourth economic skill of providers should be the awareness of the incentives which every system of organisation and financing imparts to them to direct the care delivery process in specific ways, together with the ability to look more closely at the incentives to which they are responding in their own work.

Physicians have, on the whole, resisted the intrusion of economics, claiming that they are exempt from such considerations due to their professional ethics and their special privileged relation with individual patients. There is, however, no conflict between patient welfare and medical ethics (as opposed to the medical code of practice which, depending on the country, either condones or opposes fee-for-service or under-the-counter payments) on the one hand and economics on the other hand (as distinct from personal economics in the sense of maximising or targeting net income at given levels of effort).

Which life to save when two or more patients claim the same drug, piece of equipment or doctor's time, is both a moral and an economic choice. If all patients were treated in the most lavish and sophisticated fashion, it would certainly mean that nutrition, sports, education or some other desirable sectors and industries were getting less than their share. For economic reasons, health conditions may increasingly have to be treated by methods which are neither technically optimal nor fully efficacious. While this argument, based on the economy as a whole, may not convince physicians, they will understand that the more time they themselves devote to a single patient the less attention they will be able to give to all their other patients. They may in this way be persuaded to understand that, for the health sector as a whole, they could be exchanging or giving up a few hundred home nursing visits, a renovated ward for the mentally handicapped or a few dozen hernia operations whenever they undertake a heart transplant, put somebody on the kidney machine or admit in a neurosurgical unit.

Health care managers and administrators

The managers of heatlh care institutions (such as hospitals, polyclinics, group practices) require not only the skill to consume health economics intelligently but also skills to perform certain economic calculations and analyses. Good managers of institutions should be able to supervise, if not actually carry out, economic appraisal and to prioritise the programmes of the institution; to identify periodically the incentives stemming from the ways in which the institution is organised, financed, managed and placed in the health system; and to encourage and elicit efficiency in the design and conduct of their internal programmes through incentives, norms, guidelines, etc.

Administrators of health departments and other public bodies at national and subnational levels should be able to create plans for the allocation of resources across a multi-institutional, multi-programme district or region; monitor the effects of such plans on the use, need, health status and expenditures of the population; enhance efficiency in the segment of the health care delivery system administered by them; compare alternative strategies for achieving health system goals; plan health promotion actions jointly with other sectors of the economy where useful; and accompany any specific policy proposal by an estimate of the distribution of gains and losses for the recipient group.

Self-defence will ultimately be the major incentive to acquire and maintain these new economic skills on the part of health care managers and administrators. In the short term, it would be useful to institute strong campaigns for persuasion and training, regular feedback of economic information to practice, and external audits that include indicators of economic performance.

The Regional Office has put the emphasis on the training of these target groups. Just being disseminated is a report on a survey of health economics training programmes in interested countries. The variety and richness of the programme has astonished even experts, and many teachers are now getting into contact. Work in progress will yield early in 1987, a manual on health economics training, which consists of learning material in five areas: health and the economy, health policy implementation, priority setting and strategy selection, harmonisation of provider and consumer interests, and equity, equality and reduction of status differentials. Illustrative material was contributed by more than 150 economist-teachers in nearly all European countries and then synthesised by selected experts and reviewed by interdisciplinary groups. Already, parts have been translated into Spanish, and the material is in use in the European Office's international training workshops on health economics.

It is hoped that the value that health economics has, in all its three aspects, in the mobilisation of resources and actions for HFA2000 can be demonstrated to health policy makers in a European Conference on Health Economics which is planned for summer 1989.

Part Two

Education and Research

10

Health Economics Research in the UK

Alan Maynard

INTRODUCTION

The task of analysing health economics research in the United Kingdom is complex because of the diversity of funding agencies and 'suppliers' of research activity. The UK Health Economics Study Group (HESG) has 154 members with widely disparate interests working in a variety of locations (a recent statement of their work can be found in Parkin and Yule, 1985). At least one in three of these researchers was trained at and/or work in the two major health economics research centres at the Universities of Aberdeen and York (a rough quick count shows 52 out of 154 researchers mentioned in HEART with links with these institutions). The other major centre of health economics research, the Economic Advisers' Office of the Department of Health, works closely with the York centre and contains people trained there.

One risk of such concentrations of activity is that its scope may be restricted by a group consensus which does not reflect the 'needs' of the UK research system. Certainly a group consensus emerged and was recognised many years ago (see e.g. Akehurst, 1980 and Hurst, 1980) by British researchers. In many ways it reflected some of the issues which emerged from US reviews of research (see e.g. Feldstein, 1974) but without the interests in insurance mechanisms and the workshop of for-profit and not-for-profit provider institutions.

The UK research concensus, as set out again so clearly in this volume by A.J. Culyer, reflects the markets generated for economic expertise by the National Health Service. The private health care sector in Britain is small and the private acute sector faces major cost containment problems with insurance cover growing slowly at 3 to

4 per cent per annum and the private sector bed stock declining in 1985 (Maynard, 1984a, 1986). This sector is unlikely to create major research initiatives in the near future unless the political consensus which maintains the NHS is reversed.

With the NHS the major focus of research it is not surprising that UK health economists have put so much effort into cost-effectiveness studies (such studies are reviewed, together with examples from abroad, by Drummond, 1981 and Drummond, Ludbrook, Lowson and Steele, 1986). Indeed with the cost pressures induced by technological (e.g. NHI scanners) and medical (e.g. AIDS) changes it is likely that this emphasis will be reinforced in future years.

Whilst this pressure has led to progress in the development and application of health status measures and the elaboration of economic evaluation techniques with the cost-utility (cost-quality adjusted life year or QALY) approach, it has not led to the production of extensive research results in some other areas identified as being in need of development by the UK research consensus nearly a decade ago (Akehurst, 1980; Hurst, 1980), in particular cost and production functions. Yet these areas are of importance for efficient functioning of the NHS and other health care systems.

Some of the factors affecting the development of UK research in health economics are explored in the first part of this chapter. In the second part of the chapter there is a review of research progress in the component parts of the analysis concerned with the economics of health and health care.

FACTORS AFFECTING THE CURRENT PATTERN OF HEALTH ECONOMICS RESEARCH IN THE UK

Who funds research?

The private sector: industry's unperceived needs

One striking characteristic of the finance of health economics research in the United Kingdom is its reliance on the public sector and private (charitable) trusts and the relative absence of finance from the private sector. The extent to which UK health economists have gained access to funding from the pharmaceutical industry or other health care suppliers is generally peripheral, personal and related to 'one-off crises' as perceived by the industries, usually in marketing their products.

118

In part this myopia and the emphasis on the short-run gain rather than the long-run strategy is a function of how these industries are regulated. For instance the 1968 UK Medicines Act obliges the pharmaceutical producers to evaluate 'safety and efficacy' in order to acquire a product licence to market their products. This legislation gives no incentive for producers to consider economic issues, let alone develop comprehensive and sophisticated measures of quality of life. However it is likely that these characteristics of the regulatory process will change.

Furthermore realisation of the marketing uses of economic and quality of life aspects of health care products is dawning slowly on producers. For instance Smith Kline have been evaluating a product for use in the arthritis and rheumatism area which may have little impact on the length of life but possibly substantial effects on the patients' quality of life. To identify the quality of life (QoL) issues they are using a research instrument developed at San Diego by Bush (e.g. Bush, Chen and Patrick, 1973).

However in all health care systems it is not merely QoL issues which are pertinent for marketing, economic issues are also of considerable importance. With cost containment policies in North America and 'efficiency savings' in the NHS, producers are having to compete more vigorously for markets. Furthermore consultants (specialists) and other health care providers are having to compete for shares of their hospital budgets. Slowly clinicians and industrial producers are realising that economic evaluation of costs and QALYs may be relevant if not essential in the longer run.

Public and not-for-profit provision

As industrial producers of health care products begin to realise the usefulness of separating short- and long-term priorities, public and trust funders of health care research, whilst in some cases recognising the problem, have yet to work out an efficient strategy.

The pressure to produce 'instant results' is very acute for the Department of Health's political masters. This pressure has manifested itself particularly with the Thatcher administration which, rather than turn to the research community for policy analysis, has increasingly resorted to private sector consultants. Expenditure by the NHS on such 'expertise' grew from about £700,000 in 1979 to over £13 million in 1985. Whilst this has led to a rapid development in the supply of these services, and some of these are of high quality, not all the 'expertise' supplied appears to have given good 'value for money'. As with economic evaluation,

119

there is a need to evaluate the evaluators, or consultants in the private sector.

Whilst the private consultancy sector has grown rapidly carrying out largely 'quick and dirty' appraisals of problems faced by agencies requiring 'instant wisdom', some fundamental problems facing all such work have not been remedied. Alan Williams in his chapter mentions one such problem: outcome measurement. Rather than direct research resources at the resolution of long-known and difficult to remedy research problems, sponsors have tended to encourage the use of scarce resources to analyse obvious policy problems with inadequate research techniques.

This outcome is produced by the fragmentation of research funding and by the separation of funding between medical and health service research (HSR). A major source of UK research funding in the area of health is the Medical Research Council (MRC) which in the past has tended to be dominated by medical researchers. The involvement of the MRC in health services research has been limited but is slowly beginning to change. Until there is a substantial change in attitudes and roles in both areas (medical and HSR) of study, the considerable scope for further mutual reinforcement of research efforts will be unexploited.

At present the Department of Health, the Medical Research Council and private trusts prioritise work in a fragmented and compartmentalised way. Whilst there is strength in some diversity, there may be some inefficiency in non-collaboration. The existing trade-off between diversity, independence and collaboration does not seem to be efficient. In particular too little effort seems to be being invested in ventures such as developing QoL measures and extending the use of econometric techniques (see below) with, *inter alia*, the extension of existing data sets. The time horizons of existing decision makers appear to be inhibiting the development and application of techniques which may take 5–10 years to yield fruit but whose products would radically change the nature and usefulness of health research, both economic and non-economic.

Who carries out health economics research?

Reference has already been made to the dominance of York and Aberdeen as the sources of health economists in the United Kingdom. Where do additions to this stock come from? The primary source is a DHSS funded masters course which exposes students with good first degrees in economics to a taught programme in economics, health economics and health services research. This course, which is run at York, provides only 6 new health economists each year for a health care system which spends in excess of £20,000 million annually.

The quantity of training in health economics offered to non-economists is very limited. The majority of medical students get little more than a few hours of exposure to economic techniques in 5 years of undergraduate training (see Spoor, Mooney and Maynard, 1986). The development at the University of Aberdeen of a health economics correspondence course for non-economists in the NHS is imaginative and is leading to increasing awareness of economic issues in the Service. However the majority of clinicians and managers in the NHS have either not been trained at all in economic techniques, or their training tends to be superficial.

This means that the 'in-house' capacity of NHS personnel is such that they are generally unable to carry out substantive economic appraisals themselves and, in many cases, are not sufficiently 'literate' in such techniques to permit them to evaluate studies with which they come in contact. If the economic 'literacy' of health service clinicians and managers is improved, and the scope for substantial investment in such skills by the NHS Training Authority is considerable, the demand for health economics research might increase. However, with the existing stock and flow of personnel into health economics, whether such a demand would generate a supply response is unclear.

At present existing centres recrui..ng health economists (whether substantive such as at York, Aberdeen or the DHSS, or 'one-off' as happens when a NHS health authority seeks to recruit a lone economist) face the problem of very few applicants for posts. The Universities and, to a lesser extent, the NHS have been unable to respond to this recruitment problem by raising the salaries of health economists because of rigidities imposed by centrally determined pay scales. Until 'imaginative' circumvention of these restraints leads to higher salaries and there are increases in the supply of trained researchers such recruitment problems may continue.

Another factor affecting the recruitment of researchers is the absence of a career structure. Outside the National Health Service, this is a product of the fragmentation of research funding and the reluctance of major funding agencies such as the DHSS and the MRC to offer some form of continuity for economists in the research system *per se*, let alone in any research institution. This leads to the recruitment and training in research techniques and practice of new graduates and their loss after 2 or 3 years to the attractions of greater security and income outside the health economics research community.

There are various ways of obviating such problems. An economics service for the National Health Service, with practitioners recruited for the service but paid for and likely to work in any one of its Regional or District agencies, could be developed to provide the economic services for the constituent authorities. Such an innovation could provide a career structure and wide scope for the application of economic analysis to problems manifesting themselves at all levels of the NHS. Such an organisation is being developed on a limited basis from York, the York Health Economics Consortium, which will provide economic advice and an intelligence service to two NHS Regions and their constituent District authorities.

Overview

There are two major problems arising from the current pattern of provision of health economics research in the UK. The first is the failure to achieve an efficient balance of investment in short- ('quick and dirty') and long-term (development and application of new, e.g. QoL and QALY, and existing, e.g. econometric) activities in the application of economic analysis to health and health care. This is due to the all too slowly dissipating myopia of the private sector whose decision makers cannot perceive their own self-interest in developing and applying economics in their product areas and to the dominance of the short-term imperative and the fragmentation of decision making in the public agencies and many charitable trusts. This inefficient balance in emphasis arises from the economists' failure to convince conservative, often medically dominated sponsors who seem to be, in some cases, intimidated by and unjustifiably sceptical of the development and application of such things as quality of life measures and econometric techniques. Clearly the scope for 'evangelical sales' of the health economics approach are still considerable.

The second problem associated with health economics research in the UK is the recruitment of researchers. In part this is due to the rigidity (and inadequacy in terms of calling forth a supply of competent practitioners) of salary levels in the Universities and the NHS.

However another major problem is the absence of an established career structure either in the Universities or the NHS for health economists. Until innovatory responses to these problems are identified and implemented, the efficient development of supply of economic research in the UK health sector will be inhibited.

A REVIEW OF GAPS IN HEALTH ECONOMICS KNOWLEDGE

This review will be partial in the sense that it may be incomplete and it is the view of one person who exhibits particular prejudices and is influenced by particular events in the past. Despite these problems, hopefully it will illuminate some of the priority areas for future research effort in the UK. This process of illumination will have different emphases from those of Culyer and Williams but schematically it will be developed in the context of the Williams' diagram shown in Figure 10.1.

What influences health? (box A)

The stimulus provided to the economic analysis of the demand for health by the work of Michael Grossman (1972) was substantial and has generated both theoretical and empirical development (e.g. Muurinen, 1982). Undoubtedly work of this nature would be facilitated greatly by data about consumption and investment across the life-cycle. However, gradually economic material is being mobilised in the context of a human capital model to provide insights into the relative effects of factors such as income, education, health care, leisure habits and work practices. A lot of work remains to be done but the procession is showing interest in and a willingness to work on the problems associated with the health production function.

Whilst the users of these models seek to grapple with the impact of health care and non-health care inputs on health over the life cycle, other econometric work is beginning to illuminate the characteristics of the demand for addictive substances such as alcohol and tobacco. The work is more limited in that it is concerned with consumption habits *per se* rather than the impact of such consumption on health. However it is, none the less, of significant intellectual and policy relevance. Part of this work involves the development of established demand theory to take account of

123

Figure 10.1: The structure of the discipline of health economics

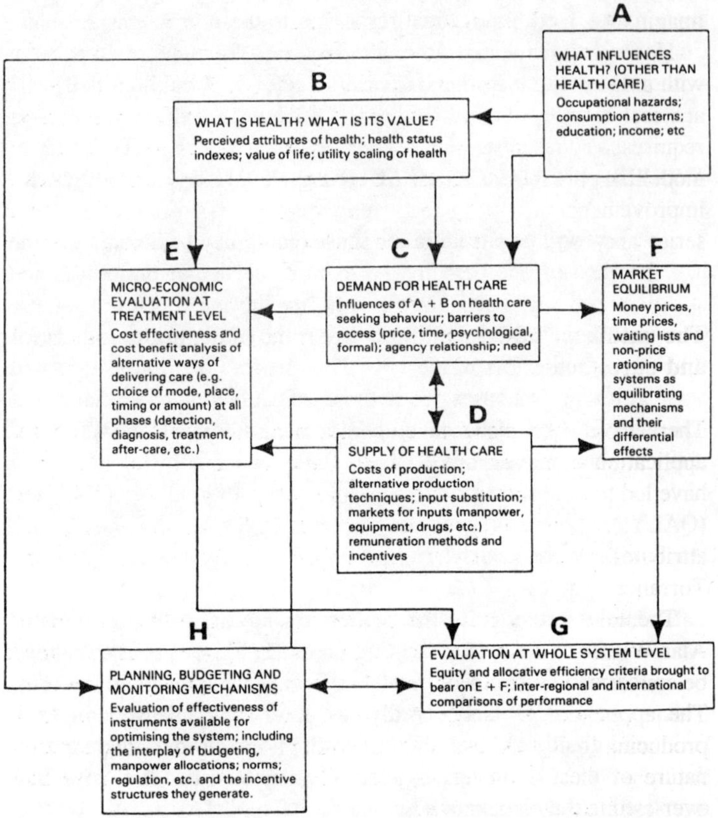

```
                                                              A
                                                    WHAT INFLUENCES
                                                    HEALTH? (OTHER THAN
                              B                     HEALTH CARE)
                                                    Occupational hazards;
            WHAT IS HEALTH? WHAT IS ITS VALUE?      consumption patterns;
            Perceived attributes of health; health status   education; income; etc
            indexes; value of life; utility scaling of health


      E                           C                              F
   MICRO-ECONOMIC          DEMAND FOR HEALTH CARE        MARKET
   EVALUATION AT           Influences of A + B on health care   EQUILIBRIUM
   TREATMENT LEVEL         seeking behaviour; barriers to   Money prices,
   Cost effectiveness and  access (price, time, psychological,   time prices,
   cost benefit analysis of   formal); agency relationship; need   waiting lists and
   alternative ways of                                     non-price
   delivering care (e.g.                                   rationing
   choice of mode, place,                      D           systems as
   timing or amount) at all                                equilibrating
   phases (detection,       SUPPLY OF HEALTH CARE          mechanisms
   diagnosis, treatment,    Costs of production;           and their
   after-care, etc.)        alternative production         differential
                            techniques; input substitution;   effects
                            markets for inputs (manpower,
                            equipment, drugs, etc.)
                            remuneration methods and
                            incentives


      H                                            G
   PLANNING, BUDGETING AND        EVALUATION AT WHOLE SYSTEM LEVEL
   MONITORING MECHANISMS          Equity and allocative efficiency criteria brought to
   Evaluation of effectiveness of   bear on E + F; inter-regional and international
   instruments available for        comparisons of performance
   optimising the system; including
   the interplay of budgeting,
   manpower allocations; norms;
   regulation, etc. and the incentive
   structures they generate.
```

addiction. For instance the analysis of habit formation and the modelling of 'addiction' within the context of changing utility function and dynamic demand offers interesting possibilities for examining choice and consumption patterns in the alcohol and tobacco markets.

The second strand of this work involves econometric testing of established theories of demand. A careful review of the literature (see e.g. Godfrey, 1986) reveals that the scale and the content of research in the UK exploring price, income, advertising, health education and other elasticities is quite limited. What is required is the testing of competing models with the same data set to establish the significance and the stability of estimates over the period since, say, 1960. What the literature offers is different model specifications using different data sets and from these it is clear that much imaginative model specification and testing could be carried out.

However such addiction control policies have costs and benefits with gains in the length and quality of life (QALYs) being acquired at a cost in terms of employment and profits. To explore these issues requires, as does the testing of the Grossman model and econometric modelling of the demand for addictive substances, significant improvements in the quantity and quality of cross-section, time series and life-cycle data sets both economic and clinical.

The nature of health and micro-economic evaluation of care and cure (boxes B and F)

There have been significant developments in the elaboration and application of measures of health status and quality of life which have led to the production of measures of quality adjusted life years (QALYs). This has generated league tables of the cost-QALY attributes of competing therapies (see e.g. Williams, 1985 and Torrance, 1986).

The case for measures of outcome is set out in this volume by Alan Williams. Such advocacy has considerable merit but there must be concern about some aspects of current developments in this area. The application of crude measures such as the Rosser index is producing 'ball park' estimates of QALYs and although the tentative nature of these estimates is generally emphasised, the naïve may over-estimate their robustness.

Such measures concentrate the minds of researchers, economists and clinicians, and policy makers wonderfully but the Rosser valuations of alternative combinations of disability and distress are derived from a very small sample (70). Furthermore knowledge about the congruence of competing quality of life measures is very limited e.g. for a given patient population how do measures on the Rosser index, the Nottingham Health Profile and other measures (e.g. those of Bush in the US or Torrance in Canada) score at any one point in time and more over time?

The inherent limitations of cost-benefit and cost-effectiveness analysis arising from the absence of measures of outcome will be mitigated by future systematic developments in the measurement of the utility of health states and the creation of crude QALY measures. Indeed cost-utility analysis offers a potentially powerful tool for the identification of the cost-QALY characteristics of competing therapies if quality of life measures are developed and applied sensibly.

As Williams argues so lucidly in this volume the need to explore these and related issues are urgent and could, if resolved, transform the nature of health economics research over the last decade. In the meantime there is a significant risk that if funders do not finance this work efficiently its policy clients may become disillusioned, particularly if conflicting results arise from different measures of the quality of life.

The demand for health care and market equilibrium (boxes C and F)

In a health care system with few price barriers to consumption, and most of these being in the public rather than the fully reimbursing private system, it is not surprising that the volume of econometric work in the UK is limited. Lavers (1983) and O'Brien (1982) have explored the price elasticity of pharmaceutical charges in the NHS but little work has been done in the market for dental services where the use of co-payments is extensive. In part this problem is a reflection of the reluctance of Government agencies to provide these data for researchers.

The extent to which researchers have explored non-price rationing devices is very limited. Whilst Culyer and Cullis (1976) have initiated some research in this area their cue has led to no further responses in terms of investigation of how markets clear in the absence of prices. The costs and benefits of these rationing devices also await analysis.

The effects of these rationing devices contribute towards the established but still under-researched social/income/class profiles inherent in the utilisation of health care and health outcomes in the UK (see e.g. the Black Report, Department of Health and Social Security, 1980 and Le Grand, 1982). The influence of unemployment on health and health care utilisation both in total and by class (interest) group is another area in need of further work (Gravelle, 1984) although such work can only be facilitated by the collection of better data sets on which to model the complex two-way interactions of health and unemployment.

126

The supply of health care (box D)

The need for more extensive analysis of cost and health care production functions has been established for over a deciade, being mentioned in the surveys cited at the beginning of this chapter. However progress with this work has been less than spectacular in the UK.

With some notable exceptions (e.g. Hurst, 1977 and Lavers and Whynes, 1978), health economists have generally ignored the opportunities to analyse with econometric techniques the supply side of the NHS. Thus despite the pioneering work of Martin Feldstein (1967) in this area, little is known about the nature of such crucial planning issues as substitution possibilities.

Looking at the broader aspects of such work and including the US literature, it is apparent that the scale of such work across the profession is limited. Furthermore that work which has been done has used different formulations of production functions (e.g. CES) and come to differing conclusions. For instance Reinhardt's (1974) analysis of ambulatory care identified the scope for the efficient substitution of doctors by nurse practitioners. Pauly's (1980) analysis of hospital production functions led to the conclusion that it would be efficient to substitute more doctors for less nurses. These results are for different health care sectors but they may be a product of this or model specification. What is needed is more work in this area using common data stocks to determine whether, for instance, the conclusions are responsive to model specification (e.g. alternative formulations of production functions).

Such work would inform manpower forecasting. At present the techniques used both in the UK and abroad are simplistic. In the UK medical manpower planning means physician manpower planning and until recently this consisted of point estimates of future stocks with no analysis of substitution possibilities or resource consequences (for a critique and elaboration see e.g. Maynard and Walker, 1977, 1978). Even though some of these defects are being remedied, manpower forecasting in the market for nurses, whose cost represents over 35 per cent of NHS expenditure, is still noticeable by its absence.

The absence of research is also noticeable for the pharmaceutical industry. The industry is very much a creature of the Government whose legislation and rules influence safety, efficacy, prices and profits. Because of competition it is not easy for researchers to acquire systematic data about the industry but even that which is

127

available would be amenable to analysis if researchers were interested in this part of the health care market. With some exceptions (e.g. Maynard, 1984b) they are not, despite the scope for the application of the economic theories of regulation and public choice and the routine analysis of the behaviour of pharmaceutical firms, using standard concepts in industrial economics.

Evaluation of the health care system and its optimisation (boxes G and H)

The evaluation of the performance of some parts of the NHS is very superficial and nowhere is this more evident than in primary care. Despite avowals by interest groups that the UK system of primary care is the 'best in the world' and 'cost-effective', the fact of the matter is that it is a black box of largely unknown content (Dowson and Maynard, 1985; Maynard, 1985; Gravelle, Marinker and Maynard, 1986a, b, c). The limited (small sample) studies that are available indicate large variations in practice with, for instance, surprisingly low patient contact hour scores and wide variations in hospital referral patterns (see e.g. Acheson, 1985).

The absence of systematic appraisal of process or health care activity is also evident in the hospital sector. Although John Yates at the University of Birmingham and the DHSS are now providing some useful computerised data on hospital staffing and some processes of care, there are still major areas of hospital process for which there are data but which are not reviewed routinely. For instance the variations in post-operative mortality between surgeons appears to be considerable from the crude data available. Little effort has yet been applied to the evaluation of whether there is a scale of activity-mortality rate e.g. do those surgeons who use a procedure rarely kill more of those patients than those surgeons who are more active in using a particular technique (i.e. are there mortality economies of scale). Such issues are beginning to be discussed (e.g. the Association of Surgeons and the Association of Anaesthetists are investigating in 5 pilot areas the circumstances surrounding all post-operative surgical deaths within 30 days and feeding back these data to consultants).

Any attempt to optimise the system of health care in the UK requires systematic data about costs, processes and outcomes (e.g. QALYs). Such data would facilitate the analysis of cost and patient shifting at the margins of the NHS. One consequence of the structure of the NHS is that the pattern of care is compartmentalised into hospital provision (the hospital and community health care budget (HCHS)), primary care (the Family Practitioner Services budget (FPS)), local authority social services (LASS), social security (SS), and household provision. Any service innovation, for instance the development of community care, shifts patients and costs, in the case of the development of community care from the cash limited HCHS budget onto the cash limited LASS budget and the open-ended (demand determined) FPS, SS and household budgets.

Such shifts may take place for reasons of financial (financial cost minimising to the institution) expediency rather than because of the adoption of efficient (opportunity cost minimising to society) policies. Indeed managers in hospitals can and do shift patients and costs onto other NHS sections often with little regard to opportunity cost and outcomes. The incentive structures are perverse in that the 'actors' in the NHS are given signals which induce often vigorous but inefficient action (for an analysis of these perverse price indicators in the field of care of the elderly, see Maynard and Smith, 1984).

The nature of these perverse incentives is not well understood and requires research involving carefully evaluated trials (RCTs) to determine efficient practices. However the identification of such practices is only a part of the solution to the problems associated with optimising the system. What is also required is new budgeting arrangements so that the managers of the compartments of the NHS can 'trade' patients and budgets as they move the pattern of care towards greater efficiency. Such arrangements can be concep- tualised (Maynard, 1984b) but are difficult to implement for historical and political reasons.

However without trials to determine the effects of new budgeting arrangements and similar work to identify efficient patterns of care it will be difficult to optimise the system of health care in the UK. At present there is continuous innovation and experimentation taking place within and between the component parts of the NHS. Unfor- tunately these 'experiments' are *ad hoc*, poorly structured and rarely evaluated. Until this inefficiency is remedied, system optimisation will be difficult to identify let alone achieve.

Such optimisation will have to consider not only efficiency issues but the explicit equity goals inherent in the design of the NHS. Consequently in evaluating the efficiency of potential service innovations such as health maintenance organisations (HMOs) the impact on minority groups and poor consumers requires careful measurement. The latter have been shown by the work of the Rand Corporation (Ware *et al.*, 1986) to offer care inferior to that of the fee per item of service system for those who are both ill and poor. This inferiority is shown in terms of both mortality and morbidity patterns measured by a variety of length and quality of life approaches.

Another aspect of the equity goals and performance of the NHS is the limited economic analysis of the budget formulae used to determine the allocation of cash limit hospital (HCHS) budgets. For instance there are considerable differences in the recourse endowments of the constituent parts of the United Kingdom with Scotland getting 17 per cent above target allocation and Northern Ireland a 20 per cent excess (Birch and Maynard, 1986 forthcoming). This problem is long identified (see Maynard and Ludbrook, 1980) but like the omission of primary care and social services expenditure from the formula approach no remedies have been implemented. Indeed after the 1976 implementation of the formula the economists have been noticeably inactive in their analysis of the existing formulae and their emendation. The Government's reappraisal of the English (RAWP) formula in 1986 may precipitate much needed new work in this area. Such equity issues and more generally the public-private mix for health care are notable in that existing stock of knowledge about 'system' performance is incomplete to a significant degree (McLachlan and Maynard, 1982).

OVERVIEW

The scope for research in health economics in the UK is very wide and involves the application of established methods (e.g. the application of the econometric techniques to the analysis of cost and production functions) and the development of new approaches (e.g. measuring the quality of life and generating estimates of the costs and quality adjusted life years (QALYs) produced by competing health and health care investments).

The development of the sub-discipline of health economics over the last 20 years has been uneven and influenced strongly by the personalities involved and their interests. Another strong influence on research development has been its funding which seems, partly because of policy pressures and partly because of its compartmentalisation, to have emphasised the short term and placed too little emphasis on the systematic development and application of, for instance, outcome measures. Furthermore these funding agencies, and the Universities have failed to create and maintain with an efficient career structure and an adequate supply of research manpower. Such problems will not go away and it is to be hoped that their recognition will lead to an evolving process of change which will ensure that knowledge is increased and the efficiency with which the NHS budget is spent is improved.

REFERENCES

Acheson, D. (1985) 'Variations in hospital referrals'. In G. Teeling-Smith (ed.), *Health, education and general practice*. Office of Health Economics, London.

Akehurst, R.L. (1980) *The social science implications of the report of the Royal Commission on the National Health Service: an economists view*. Unpublished mimeograph, University of York.

Birch, S. and Maynard, A. (1986) 'The RAWP review: Rawping primary care and Rawping the United Kingdom'. *Centre for Health Economics Discussion Paper* no. 19, University of York.

Bush, J.W., Chen, M.M. and Patrick, D.L. (1973) 'Health status index in cost effectiveness: analysis of a PKU program'. In R.L. Berg (ed.), *Health status indexes*. Hospital Research and Education Trust, Chicago.

Culyer, A.J. and Cullis, J. (1976) 'Some economics of hospital waiting lists in the NHS'. *Journal of Social Policy, 4*.

Department of Health and Social Security (1980) *Inequalities in health*. A report chaired by Sir Douglas black (the Black Report), HMSO, London.

Dowson, S. and Maynard, A. (1985) 'General practice'. In A. Harrison and J. Gretton (eds), *Health care 1985*. CIPFA, London.

Drummond, M.F. (1981) *Studies in economic appraisal in health care*. Oxford University Press, Oxford.

────── Ludbrook, A., Lowson, K. and Steele, A. (1986) *Studies in economic appraisal in health care*, Vol. 2. Oxford University Press, Oxford.

Feldstein, M. (1976) *Economic analysis for health service efficiency*. North Holland, Amsterdam.

────── (1974) 'Econometric studies in health care'. In M. Intriligator and D.A. Kendrick (eds), *Priorities of quantitative economics*, Vol. 2. North Holland, Amsterdam.

Godfrey, C. (1986) 'Factors influencing the consumption of alcohol and tobacco: a review of demand models'. *Centre for Health Economics, Discussion Paper*, University of York.

Gravelle, H. (1984) 'Does unemployment kill?' *Nuffield-York Portfolio Series, Folio 9*, Nuffield Provincial Hospitals Trust, London.

────── Marinker, M. and Maynard, A. (1986a) 'The doctor, the patient and their contract: the GPs contract why change it?' *British Medical Journal, 292*, 1313–15 (17 May).

———— Marinker, M. and Maynard, A. (1986b) 'The doctor, the patient and their contract: a good practice allowance: is it feasible?' *British Medical Journal, 292*, 1374–76 (24 May).

———— Marinker, M. and Maynard, A. (1986c) 'The doctor, the patient and their contract: alternative contracts: are they viable?' *British Medical Journal, 292* (31 May).

Grossman, M. (1972) *The demand for health: a theoretical and empirical investigation*. National Bureau of Economic Research, University of Chicago Press, Chicago.

Hurst, J. (1977) *Saving hospital expenditure by reducing in-patient stay*. Government Economic Services, HMSO, London.

———— (1980) *Research priorities for health economics in the 1980s: a tentative strategy*. Economic Advisers Office, Department of Health and Social Security (unpublished).

Lavers, R.J. (1983) 'The effects of price changes on the demand for and cost of pharmaceutical prescriptions, 1970–81'. Paper presented to the International Conference on Health Economics, Lille, France, September.

———— and Whynes, D. (1978) 'A production function analysis of English maternity hospitals'. *Socio-Economic Planning Sciences, 12*, 2.

Le Grand, J. (1982) *The strategy of equality*. Allen and Unwin, London.

Maynard, A. (1984a) 'Private practice: answer or irrelevance'. *British Medical Journal, 288*, 1849–51.

———— (1984b) 'Budgeting in health care systems'. *Effective Health Care, 2*, 2, 41–50.

———— (1985) 'Performance incentives'. In G. Teeling-Smith (ed.), *Health, education and general practice*. Office of Health Economics, London.

———— (1986) 'Public and private sector interactions: an economic perspective'. *Social Science and Medicine, 22*.

———— and Ludbrook, A. (1980) 'Applying the resource allocation formula to the constituent parts of the UK'. *Lancet*, i.

———— and Smith, J. (1984) 'The elderly: who cares? who pays?' *Nuffield-York Portfolio Series, Folio 1*, Nuffield Provincial Hospitals Trust, London.

———— and Walker, A. (1977) 'Too many doctors?' *Lloyds Bank Review, 125*.

———— and Walker, A. (1978) 'Doctor manpower 1975–2000: alternative forecasts and their resource implications'. *Royal Commission on the National Health Service, research paper, no. 4*. HMSO, London.

McLachlan, G. and Maynard, A. (eds) (1982) *The public private mix for health*. Nuffield Provincial Hospitals Trust, London.

Muurinen, J.M. (1982) 'Demand for health: a generalised model'. *Journal of Health Economics, 1*, 1, 5–28.

O'Brien, B. (1982) 'The demand for prescriptions: dispensing with charges'. Paper presented to the Health Economists Study Group, Brunel University.

Parkin, D. and Yule, B. (1985) *Health economists activities, research and training*, (HEART). Centre for Health Economics, University of York (this publication is revised annually).

Pauly, M. (1980) *Doctors and their workshops: economic models of physician behavior*. National Bureau of Economic Research, University of Chicago Press, Chicago.

Reinhardt, U.E. (1974) *Physician productivity and the demand for health manpower*. Ballinger, Cambridge, Massachusetts.

Spoor, C., Mooney, G. and Maynard, A. (1986) 'Teaching health economics'. *British Medical Journal, 292,* 785.

Torrance, G.W. (1986) 'Measurement of health state utilities for economic appraisal: a review'. *Journal of Health Economics, 5,* 1–300.

Wagstaff, A. (1986) 'The demand for health: some new empirical evidence'. *Journal of Health Economics, 5,* 3, 195–233.

Ware, J., Brook, R., Rogers, W.H., Keeler, E.B., Davies, A., Sherbourne, G., Goldberg, G.A., Camp, P. and Newhouse, J.P. (1986) 'Health insurance: comparison of health outcomes at Health Maintenance Organisation with those of fee per item of service care'. *Lancet, 8488,* 1, 1017–22 (3 May).

Williams, A. (1985) 'Economics of coronary artery bypass grafting'. *British Medical Journal, 291,* 326–9 (3 August).

11

Future Directions in Health Economics Research in the USA

Gail Wilensky

Predicting the future is always a high risk venture, whether it is the future of health policy, the future of health economics research or the future production of health economists. In trying to predict future directions, I have found it helpful to review the course of health economics over the past twenty years.

PAST AS PROLOGUE TO THE FUTURE

The most significant change in health economics over the past two decades was the application of modern quantitative economic techniques, beginning in the late 1960s. The result of this change has been the movement of health economics in the United States from an era dominated by institutional economists and a primary focus on the institutions associated with the financing and delivery of health care, to an era dominated by economists trained in modern micro-economic theory and econometrics. The individual most responsible for this change was Martin Feldstein beginning with his seminal piece on hospital cost functions (Feldstein, 1967).

What is clear in reviewing the focus of research in health economics over the past few decades is that health economics is an area where research follows policy. Thus, predicting the future of health economic research, means predicting the future of health policy. The key policy issues addressed by health economics research since the late 1960s have been access to health care, the sensitivity of demand to price and income, the behaviour of physicians and hospitals within the context of micro-economic theory, and cost containment. The list of the publications concerning the utilisation of health services by the poor and minority populations relative to other populations, estimates of price and income elasticities in the demand for medical care, theories and empirical estimates of hospital behaviour, and physician-induced demand, could occupy the remainder of this paper. Ironically, society's success in coping with these issues has itself created new problems that will dominate health economics in the 1980s and 1990s.

FUTURE DIRECTIONS IN HEALTH POLICY

What are these future directions in health policy? They are, not surprisingly, the logical extensions of where we are now. That is: the movement to managed care, payment reform, quality in an era of cost containment and managed care, the uninsured in a competitive environment, for-profit versus not-for-profit delivery systems, the impact of the changing physician supply and an ageing population.

Managed care

The adoption of a prudent buyer mentality with its focus on value for the health care dollar, combined with the decline in cost based reimbursement, has spawned the managed care movement. Managed care comes in many forms — Health Maintenance Organisations (HMOs), Individual Practice Associations (IPAs), Preferred Provider Organisations (PPOs), Primary Care Networks (PCNs), case managers, etc. — and varies from the extremely restrictive to the minimally restrictive. The common element is management of the way the patient interacts with providers and the placement of providers at some degree of financial risk in terms of the resources used by the patients.

There are a series of research questions which will be raised by this shift to managed care. These include: the characteristics of the individuals who choose managed care, an analysis of why some individuals choose various types of managed care, the implications of various types of managed care on the cost of delivering care and the mix of resources used in delivering that care. These questions have all been raised in the research directed towards Health Maintenance Organisations. That research is as yet incomplete and will become subsequentially more complicated by all of the variants on managed care. An additional issue which has been of fundamental

135

importance to all forms of managed care is biased selection. A recent review of that literature (Wilensky and Rossiter, 1986) indicates that the issue of biased selection is far from settled.

Although the rise in managed care represents one of the most significant changes in health care delivery, there has been little research on this subject to date. There are basically two reasons for this. First, we are in the middle of an enormous amount of change. It is not clear, for example, whether some of the variants of managed care, such as preferred provider organisations, are in fact different entities from individual practice associations or whether within a few years these two types of organisations will evolve into a single form. Trying to analyse change while it is still occurring is a difficult and perhaps meaningless activity. Second, there are inevitable lags in data availability. Although research in health economics is frequently data-dependent, this is particularly true with regard to managed care.

Payment reform

Policy makers in the 1980s have been forced to cope with a clash of opposite forces as never before. On the one hand, there is strong political demand in the United States to contain and even reduce federal government spending relative to Gross National Product (GNP). On the other hand, there is also growing demand for broader and deeper Medicare coverage for the aged. Furthermore, even if Medicare coverage did not change, Medicare outlays would still continue to exceed revenues by ever growing amounts.

Faced with the necessity of reconciling opposing political forces, policy makers have turned to Medicare payment system reform in an attempt to extract from providers more and better health care for the dollar. The first step occurred in 1983 with the introduction of prospective payment for hospitals, which established a fixed payment per diagnosis. While the results of this change are already being evaluated, researchers are also assessing more sweeping reforms. The focus of payment reform research will be on:

1. how services should be combined and how that combination should be paid for;
2. the economic implications of different ways of financing Medicare long term.

136

Quality of care

Health policy analysts have become increasingly concerned about the impact of cost containment and managed care on quality. The difficulty is that quality of care remains as elusive as ever and perhaps becomes even more difficult to measure in the face of changing delivery modes. Measuring quality of care as process, that is, defining quality in terms of whether particular procedures have been followed for given symptoms, has never been very satisfactory; it would be particularly misleading, however, given the change which is occurring in the way the care is being organised and delivered. The primary alternative to process, however, is outcome and, at least historically, measuring clinical outcomes as a result of differing delivery strategies has been both rare and costly.

While the importance of quality as a major issue is well accepted, the role of the economist in analysing the issue is less clear. Traditionally, economists have not dealt with quality but there seems to be a growing sense that analysing the impact of cost containment and managed care without explicit recognition of its potential impact on quality is no longer meaningful.

The uninsured in a competitive environment

The problems of the uninsured and of uncompensated medical care have been the most visible negative consequence of the movement to a more competitive health care environment in the United States. The care of the uninsured and the underinsured has traditionally been financed implicitly, that is, by cross subsidy. In an era of prudent buyer behaviour, care which used to be financed implicitly has now been placed at risk. This does not really represent a new direction in health economic research; it is rather the re-emergence of access as an issue in health care delivery. In the short-term, at least, we can expect to see continued interest in the numbers of uninsured people in the United States, the impact of their lack of coverage on the utilisation of health services and perhaps on health status and their impact on the provider community.

For-profit versus not-for-profit delivery systems

There has been substantial interest and concern about the impact of the increasing role of for-profit delivery systems in health care. Like the access issue, this is not really a new area of research but an extension of research concerning the behaviour of the physician and the hospital. There continues to be substantial debate about the impact of for-profit hospitals on cost and quality of care and it can be expected that this will lead to continued empirical analyses of this issue. As many analysts have already noted, however, the issue appears to be more a matter of multi-hospital systems versus single hospitals than it does for-profit versus not-for-profit since many not-for-profit chains have for-profit subsidiaries. It is, therefore, more likely that much of the future research will centre on the impact of the multi-hospital system and the multi-dimensional health care system as opposed to the more current fascination with the difference between for-profit and not-for-profit delivery systems. This is an additional area in which data needs will keep us behind the times.

Changing physician supply

Analysis of physician behaviour has long been a mainstay of health economic research. While some aspects of physician behaviour have already received extensive attention, such as physician-induced demand, the substantial increase in physician supply which will occur over the next decade will rekindle interest in physician behaviour. Among the research issues which are likely to be addressed and readdressed are the impact of increasing physician supply on health care expenditures, physician-induced demand, and the adoption of alternative delivery systems. The most important aspects of this additional research are not likely to occur for another 5–10 years, given the expected increases in physician supply over time and the subsequent lags in the availability of relevant data.

The ageing of the population

While the impact of the ageing of the population on the health care system will be profound, the impact of health economics research in the next 10–20 years will be relatively small. The reason is two-fold. First, the major impact of the ageing of the population will not occur for another 20 years. Second, and probably more important, the impact of ageing *per se* will be more the topic of demographers and gerontologists, rather than health economists. The main health economics issue raised by the ageing of the population will be how to finance the care of the elderly, and how to structure the payment and delivery systems for long-term care as well as acute care.

Methodological trends in health economics research

The use of econometrics and micro-economic theory to predict behaviour of providers and consumers has been a major part of health economics research for much of the last two decades. I expect the increased use of econometrics and the increased interest of econometricians in health care to continue. This should be particularly true for analyses of treatment variations, length of stay and cost analyses associated with various types of managed care. The sustained rate of increase in expenditures makes these issues of continuing interest to policy makers; the availability of large data sets will make these areas attractive to econometricians and will also probably result in elaborate econometric models. At the same time, there is likely to be a new-found interest in the use of case studies and other methods of industrial organisation analysis. The movement toward vertical and horizontal integration, implied by the continuing development of multi-hospital systems and multi-dimension health care systems, as well as other components of market structure and industry structure can best be understood through traditional case study analyses. This is an area of economics which previously has been untapped in health economics and it has been rare that individuals with industrial organisation backgrounds have gone into health economics research. This is likely to change in the future.

THE TEACHING OF HEALTH ECONOMICS

There are at least two relevant dimensions regarding the future teaching of health economics: where will future health economists be trained and where will the teaching of health economics occur? Once again the past serves as a useful predictor of the future. Over the past two decades, most health economists have come from one of two roots. A small number have been trained as health economists while in graduate school. The majority of economists currently doing research in health economics, however, were trained as public finance economists or labour economists and became interested in health sometime during their career. Occasionally, this was a result of a dissertation in health economics or work as a research assistant on a health economics project but frequently it occurred at a later point in the economist's career as well. These two entry routes will continue in the future. A small number of institutions in the United States have a sufficient interest in the economics department to have health economics offered as a field of study. Just as Martin Feldstein at Harvard University trained a number of the current health economists, so will his students and others provide a number of economists specifically trained in the area of health economics. The larger number of economists who work in health, however, are likely to be individuals trained in public finance and labour who apply their discipline training to the health area. A final source of health economists/health service researchers will be trained by health economists who have appointments in health service research centres and schools of public health. The individuals thus trained, however, will have only a limited background in economics.

While the training of health economists is likely to continue to be in economics departments, the placement of health economists and the teaching of health economics will frequently occur in other settings. Casual observation in the United States makes it clear that departments of health service research and public health schools have become increasingly attractive settings for individuals interested in health economics. While some of these individuals have joint appointments in the departments of economics of their universities, their prime affiliation is the health services research centre, school of public health or medical school. This will probably continue in the future. There is no indication that economics departments are likely to regard health economics as a separate and legitimate field of study the way they do, for example, labour, public finance, industrial organisation, etc.

The placement of health economists in centres of health services research or schools of public health will impact the teaching of health economics as well. There is likely to continue to be some demand for health economics at an undergraduate level in the economics department as long as there are health economists who are affiliated with the economics departments at the universities. The availability of health economics at the graduate level will be much more sporadic and is likely to represent a single course rather than a sequence of courses at the graduate level. An increasing area of demand will be in the PhD programmes in health services research with health economics being taught to people with professional training rather than economists *per se*. While the health services research centres and schools of public health with a major orientation to health economics will be a primary site of placement for health economists and a secondary producer of quasi-economic health services researchers, the field is likely to continue to be dominated by economists at least for the next decade.

CONCLUSION

The future of health economics research will follow the areas of greatest interest in health economics policy: managed care, payment reform, quality, the uninsured and access to care, for-profit versus not-for-profit providers, the changing physician supply and the aging of the population. There will be an increased commingling between health services research and health economics with health services research centres and schools of public health continuing to be the site of placement for many health economists but not the major source of contributors to the field. Given the relatively small number of places and individuals training economists with a particular interest in health, it is likely that the shortage of well trained health economists will continue in the future.

ACKNOWLEDGEMENT

I am grateful to Mark Pauly of the University of Pennsylvania, Randall Ellis of Boston University, Stephen Long of the Congressional Budget Office, and Samuel Mitchell of the Federation of American Health Systems for sharing their thoughts with me about future directions in health economics research.

REFERENCES

Feldstein, M. (1967) *Economic analysis for health services efficiency: econometric studies of the British National Service*. North Holland, Amsterdam.
Wilensky, G. and Rossiter, L. (1986) 'Patient self selection in HMOs'. *Health Affairs*, 5, 1.

141

12

Developments in the Teaching of Health Economics: Education, Training and Evangelism

Martin Buxton

INTRODUCTION

In health economics, as in most professions, teaching is not the glamorous and prestigious activity. It is research that generally attracts both professional and lay attention, and teaching goes relatively unnoticed (except, one hopes, by those being taught). But, again like any profession, if health economics is to continue to thrive and to build on developments of the past twenty years and to carry out research that is academically strong, relevant to policy problems and likely to be considered in decision making, then teaching must play its part. It may be useful to distinguish three essential roles. Firstly, it has to provide a rigorous *education* for the next generation of professional health economists, not simply reproducing clones of the existing human capital stock but hopefully evolving a stronger breed even more appropriate to the environment in which they will work. It should also provide a *training* in some of the basic skills of health economics for those with other professional backgrounds, who need (and have recognised their need) to be able to use and understand the analytical tools and frameworks of health economics alongside their other management or planning skills. And finally teaching needs, in a rather evangelistic way, to generate *understanding* and *appreciation* of the role, actual and potential, of health economics amongst those who are rarely likely to use the techniques directly but who play crucial roles in health care — particularly the professional care-givers, clinicians and nurses — who are directly instrumental in many of the major economic decisions in health care.

This chapter illustrates what is happening with respect to these three aspects of teaching by reference to a number of recent initiatives principally in the UK. It goes on to consider some of the future changes and challenges which may have relevance not just for the UK but to health economics worldwide.

WHAT IS HEALTH ECONOMICS?

As part of the process of developing a professional identity, of clarifying a role, and giving their product an identity, health economists have from time to time attempted systematically to define and delinate what health economics is or is not.

Alan Williams (1979) made the distinction between an 'area of study' or *topic* and a 'mode of thinking' or *discipline*. The contrast is between a set of phenomena that exists to be studied and the conceptual and analytical framework for studying it. In these terms health economics is not a discipline in its own right distinct from that of economics: as has been pointed out 'there are few techniques of economic analysis that are not applicable in the topic of health; moreover there are few theoretical ideas in health economics that are truly *sui generis*' (Culyer, 1981, p. 4). Nor is it a clearly defined topic in its own right — it has no conceptual boundaries other than those of the topic 'health'. The bounds of current research for example are fairly arbitrary, differ from one country to another and in no sense represent agreed and maintainable boundaries. Thus the accepted view is to define health economics as the discipline of economics applied to the topic health. The importance of this is quite simple — it emphasises that for an economist or student of economics, health is one of many possible areas in which to apply economics. For those concerned professionally with the topic of health and the problems within it, economics is one of many possible disciplines to apply to them.

There are no clear boundaries to the topic of health but two issues are perhaps worth noting. The first has been raised on a number of occasions, namely that most health economics should better be described as health care economics. Much of the research and teaching concerns the *relatively* confined field of health care rather than the much broader topic of health. Certainly the focus of this chapter, the book as a whole, the work of OHE and probably the bulk of professional economics research and teaching on health is related to health care, its formal and informal structure, its allocation problems etc. *Relatively* little attention has been paid to the broader issues of the determinants of health, the way industrial structure affects health, although these have not been totally neglected.

The second issue concerns the balance within health (care) economics between 'macro' issues such as the organisation of health care systems, of aggregate levels of spending on health care and 'micro' issues such as the economic evaluation of therapies and technologies, resource allocation within specific budgets, and of incentive systems. Both areas are important in teaching but views about their relative importance differ.

EDUCATION OF UNDERGRADUATE AND GRADUATE ECONOMISTS

The preceding apparent digression into defining health economics is highly pertinent to an understanding of what is, and should be, taught to different groups. For undergraduates, particularly those specialising in economics, most courses in applied economics are offered to provide illustrations of the way economic theory can be used in practical contexts. Such teaching often relies on simplified examples, drawn from actual practical applications or applied research, and therefore as a teaching vehicle the value of the applied areas increases with the extent of actual use of, and research into, the discipline applied to the topic. For most undergraduate purposes, the application is secondary to the theory or analytical framework being applied and courses tend to be rather divorced from institutional and policy reality. It is interesting to note how a recently published *general* introductory economics text (Culyer, 1985) makes extensive use of health related applications as brief examples and illustrative case studies. This is, of course, in part a reflection of the interests of the author, but it is also a reflection of the extent to which economics applied to health care is now accepted as part of the mainstream of applied economics.

The exact number of undergraduate courses specifically concerned with health economics being taught varies from year to year. In a number of universities a course may have a major health component but cover other areas of social policy. However information from a survey carried out by Hersh-Cochran (1986) and more up-to-date knowledge of a number of universities suggests that there are in the UK at least a dozen undergraduate courses with a significant health economics component.

By comparison there are very few postgraduate degree courses in the UK in which health economics figures as a major element. Indeed the MSc course at the University of York is the only taught

Masters course specifically on health economics. The UK situation contrasts with that in the USA and in Canada where, from the evidence of the survey by Hersh-Cochran, the majority of teaching of health economics is at a postgraduate level. The York one-year postgraduate course was set up in 1977 with the support of the DHSS, who fund six studentships through the Economics and Social Research Council. The objectives of the course are:

> to train competent general economists who are conversant with the literature in the health and personal social services field, are capable of collaborating intelligently with other professionals in the field and are fully initiated into empirical research at the grass-roots level (Centre for Health Economics, 1985).

The course consists of two parts — a taught and examined course over two terms covering four fields of study and two to three months practical project work leading to a short dissertation. The taught courses are (1) mathematics and econometrics; (2) micro- and macro-economic theory; (3) health economics and (4) aspects of medical sociology, epidemiology, clinical research and evaluation. This course requires a very sound undergraduate training in economics, and, as can be seen even from the course titles, focuses very much on developing rigorous analytical skills and a deeper understanding of economic theory with a particular focus on health economics. It is as much about developing students understanding of the discipline as their ability to apply it to the health field. It has provided a small, but important, flow of new entrants to health economics research, who have helped to cope with the growth in the commitment of the research community. However an output of six UK students per year (plus a similar number of overseas students) can hardly hope in itself to have much impact on the supply to the NHS of personnel with specific training in health economics.

The result of the combined undergraduate and postgraduate situations is that there is still a relatively small output of economists whose formal university training will have included a substantive element of health economics. And in the foreseeable future in the UK, the contraction of the university sector is likely to lead to rationalisation of courses and a reduction in applied options such as those in health economics unless, as is the case at Brunel University, externally-funded research groups can provide such teaching at no cost to the university itself.

TRAINING HEALTH SERVICE MANAGERS AND PLANNERS

If therefore, undergraduate courses by nature of their limited breadth and postgraduate degree courses by nature of their limited extent do not attempt to train potential health service managers and planners then such training must be provided, if it is to be provided at all, by other routes.

In a survey of nearly 900 chief officers in the NHS, 'economic aspects of health' was ranked second (to personal and interpersonal skills) out of nine knowledge areas and skills in terms of the officers assessments of their personal need for further education and training (Dixon and de Metz, 1982). In the light of this survey, and greatly influenced by the Thwaites Report (Thwaites, 1977) which argued the case for a high level management development programme specifically aimed at the most senior health service managers, the King's Fund College in London set up the Corporate Management Programme (CMP). This has a modular structure, a health service focus, a chief officer target group and as yet a non-qualification based status. From the outset, this programme has contained a significant element of health economics — initially as an option in its own right, and more recently as part of a compulsory module on analytical methods. However in this, and other such courses, the emphasis on 'management development' is increasingly being taken to imply a concentration of issues of *management* approaches, techniques and styles, rather than on the concepts and techniques of the analytical *disciplines*.

Aiming rather more at middle management in the NHS (as well as medical and nursing staff), the Health Economics Research Unit at the University of Aberdeen has run correspondence courses in Health Economics each year since 1978/79. These now take about 120 students a year in the UK (and is also run in Denmark and Ireland). The objective of the courses is stated as being:

> not to convert students into amateur economists; rather it is to indicate what economics in health care is about and its strengths (and weaknesses) in assisting health care planning and evaluation. As such it is attempting to influence the thinking of students regarding how to approach problems of resource allocation in health care (University of Aberdeen, 1986).

These, and a number of other initiatives, each make a contribution to the appreciation of the role of economics in health care, and to creating a body of managers able to utilise the basic economic concepts and analytical frameworks. However, whether they be the high-flyers of the CMP, or the committed enthusiasts taking correspondence courses, there is a tendency for these courses to appeal to the already converted rather than to make new converts. And, in almost all of these initiatives, there is a disappointing lack of involvement of clinicians and nurses.

EVANGELISM: CONVERTING CLINICIANS

A number of initiatives in teaching health economics in the UK have in recent years been directed specifically towards clinicians, not in any expectation of turning them into health economists but in the hope of providing them with an appreciation of what economics is about, and why and how it is relevant to them professionally. Whether this activity should most correctly be termed as education, teaching, or evangelism is debateable. Much of it is as much about changing attitudes as imparting new information or skills. It is seen as an essential stepping-stone to gaining more widespread acceptance of the ideas, methodology and analytical framework of health economics in clinical matters.

In practice, many of the *ad hoc* initiatives would not be necessary if the medical profession had followed the advice of its own leaders about curricula within Medical Schools. The General Medical Council published in 1980 its recommendations concerning basic medical education, which asserted that: 'the necessary understanding of medicine as an evolving discipline must be attached through the study of the physical, biological, behavioural and social sciences and by the study of man himself in health and disease' (General Medical Council, 1980, p. 1). In addition to this general inclusion by implication of health economics under the cloak of social sciences as a whole, the Education Committee of the GMC specifically recommended that the teaching of Community (Social and Preventive) Medicine should include 'simple health care economics' (GMC, 1980, p. 23).

However, a survey of medical schools carried out in 1985 found that of 26 schools providing the necessary information 'six had no undergraduate programme whatsoever in health economics; and about three quarters of those which did provide instruction, devoted four hours or less of each student's entire undergraduate career to the subject' (Spoor, Mooney and Maynard, 1986). The thirteen postgraduate courses provided a rather better picture in that all included the topic but still only six included more than 20 hours of such teaching.

Various reasons were offered in that survey for the low extent of health economics teaching and nine schools reported that they were planning to increase their health economics over the next two to three years. A frequently expressed problem is that of pressure on the curriculum, and it is therefore interesting to note that the Education Committee of the GMC has set up a working party to look into the teaching of the behavioural sciences, community medicine, and general practice.

In the meantime, most of the training for clinicians in health economics is fairly *ad hoc*. A number of 'training courses' for clinicians are run by, or on behalf of, Regional Health Authorities, particularly targeted at senior Registrars or young consultants. This activity has been encouraged by support initially from the DHSS and subsequently NHS Training Authority, but these courses again rely on a process of self-selection that generally leaves vast numbers of clinicians completely uninvolved.

To attempt to make intellectual contact with some of these a number of articles have been published in the mainstream clinical literature, by leading exponents of health economics. For example, the *British Medical Journal* published over a period of twelve weeks in 1982/83 a series of articles by Mike Drummond and Gavin Mooney (1982–83) presenting the 'essentials of health economics'. This was very much an educational exercise rather than an attempt to present original material. The fact that the *BMJ* wanted to publish such a series is itself an important indication of a new acceptance of the relevance of the subject to clinicians. The concluding article expressed the aspirations of the series:

> As economists we try to understand the functioning of the NHS and see how economics can contribute to an equitable, efficient health service. We hope that doctors in their turn will see the value of trying to understand and apply the principles of economics in their pursuit of the same goal (Drummond and Mooney, 1983, p. 4).

A further encouraging sign is that a number of prominent clinicians have themselves been converted and turned evangelist. Howard Hiatt, Dean of the Harvard School of Public health has emphasised that clinicians need: 'to develop the skills to assess the benefits and costs of each intervention' (Hiatt, 1981, p. 259). More recently Bryan Jennett, Professor of Neurosurgery and Dean of the Faculty of Medicine at Glasgow University in one of the *British Medical Journal's* signed leading articles focused on the need for economic appraisal and concluded with the suggestion that: 'the entrepreneurial spirit associated with the clinical freedom fighters ('I know what's best for my patients regardless of trials or economics') begins to sound distinctly old fashioned' (Jennett, 1984).

THE NEXT TWENTY YEARS

The whole position of health economics has rapidly changed in the last twenty or so years, as this volume testifies. Change will continue. But two broad scenarios now seem to present themselves. The first, the optimistic one, that growth of health economics will continue, albeit perhaps at a rather steadier pace; that the impressive, if still rather patchy, achievements in research and education will be consolidated and built on, and that health economics will become a *fully* accepted part of the training and education and research armoury in health care. The second scenario, illustrates a nagging concern that perhaps we could be near to the peak of a cycle and that interest in, and enthusiasm for health economics will wane, speeded perhaps in the UK at least by an emphasis on techniques of *management* rather than on techniques of *analysis*. This cyclical view would then suggest that health economics should be seen as a passing fashion, and health economists as a professional group that in the end may be judged as having failed to deliver on their promises of better resource allocation.

The latter scenario is at least plausible and one that many of the critics of health economics have already predicted. However it is offered here not as an prediction but as a reminder of what is a fairly natural course of events — of growth and decay — unless positive steps are taken. A number of such steps particularly relating to education are set out below. They may well represent the factors that determine which scenario comes about.

(A) Future education must be able to point to the *proven* relevance and usefulness of health economics, rather than merely the putative or claimed future relevance. This achievement depends upon the efforts of the research community. A mature profession cannot continue to rely on reports that it 'shows promise' but has to make its case on actual achievements. These need to be documented — fairly and critically — and then need to be incorporated into the case material for teaching purposes. These achievements do exist (and some are referred to elsewhere in this volume) and others are on the near horizon. These applications, techniques, and results of a number of recent and on-going research projects need to be rapidly incorporated into the body of accepted knowledge and so to improve teaching material. Good up-to-date general textbooks on health economics are needed. Their absence in the UK has been a handicap, now at least partly removed by Gavin Mooney's new text (Mooney, 1986). Unfortunately the institutional specificity of such books makes it difficult readily to use good texts produced in other countries. For example for use in the UK, a text such as that of Evans (1984), despite its general excellence, is inappropriate because of its focus on the Canadian institutional framework.

(B) There needs to be an effort made to ensure that an adequate amount of top-quality teaching of health economics is incorporated into *all* undergraduate courses at *all* medical schools. This requires continued pressure on those responsible for influencing or determining curricula. Careful thought needs to be given as to which aspects of health economics should have priority within the limited time available within medical curricula. A greater emphasis needs to be given to the more directly relevant micro issues of evaluation of medical practice, technology assessment, and priorities within health care, rather than the macro issues of different types of health care systems and levels of spending. Two factors may help to encourage a little more time in the medical curricula for health economics. One is the increasing awareness of the problem of scarcity of resources for health care as compared with the range of possibilities offered by new technology and pharmaceuticals. The other is the increasing involvement of clinicians in management, in the UK particularly, under the new general management arrangements. The greater involvement of some senior clinicians may, by example, encourage the view that clinicians need to be concerned not only with the treatment of individual patients but also the evaluation and decision making that effectively determines which patients can be treated in what ways. But economists also need to arrange to overcome the problems of availability of appropriate teachers and teaching materials for health economics that were noted in the recent survey, and are cited as having hindered the expansion of teaching of the subject.

(C) A concern to focus on clinicians must not be at the expense of failing to offer teaching to other professionals. In particular nurses and paramedics have tended to be forgotten. As groups they directly account for large proportions of health care expenditure, and play a role in resource allocation that it all too often ignored or minimised. Much of the movement towards care in the community will mean that many important resource allocation decisions are removed from clinicians to community staff.

(D) Health economics has to become even more willing to work constructively with other disciplines. The current directions in research and emphasis in teaching, on benefit measurement for example, require, and should naturally lead to, an increasingly multi-disciplinary approach to health economics. The period of needing to sell economics by emphasising its differentiation from other disciplines and approaches has probably passed. There is a widespread, if still patchy, appreciation of the distinctive features and role of economics and now the emphasis needs to be more integrative. Health economics now needs to focus on how it relates to other important disciplines that can and should be applied to health care. If the interrelationships and interdependence of disciplines are not recognised, the promises of what health economics can offer are likely to become over-inflated and the inability to fulfil the promises compromised. The need, and scope, for co-operation is now recognised by some of the other relevant professional groups. For example, an internationally supported text on epidemiology concludes: 'The complementary approaches of the economist and the epidemiologist, and the obligatory cross-fertilisation of the two disciplines, provides one of the most promising features of the current scene' (Knox, 1979, p. 163). However, the passage goes on to suggest that, in health service planning the two professions do not often work together for the main reason that 'health economists are an even rarer species than epidemiologists'. As health economists have, and continue to, become less scarce the opportunities for collaborative research and teaching will need to be seized.

(E) For economics students there may be now a need to recognise that there is unlikely to be scope for much more specialised health economics teaching. Indeed a further push to the process of reintegration of the specialism into the mainstream may benefit both the broad discipline of economics and the specialist discipline of economics applied to health. There are a number of areas in which health economics has pushed the discipline forward, particularly in handling non-monetary data on benefits and relative values, which may be relevant to other applied fields. At the same time there are developments in other fields of applied economics that need to be considered in relationship to health. Increased specialism of undergraduate and graduate teaching will discourage these processes. However, if economists wishing to work in the health field are likely increasingly to be 'non-specialists', then there is a need to establish a method of rapid immersion for them into the topic of health, its institutional and political complexities, and its jargon and buzzwords. This needs to be negotiated with the health service (indeed the health care industry as a whole) and established, so that whether by on-the-job immersion or crash course, economists can be given the necessary detailed background to enable them to make full use in the health field of their skills.

These five main ideas for the future do not represent predictions or forecasts, but they are feasible steps that health economists need to consider. Without these or similar measures, the prospects may be worrying. Growth and decay is a real possibility. But with positive action there is a potentially attractive scenario of a healthy, respected, profession continuing to contribute to the benefit of the topic of health care and to the development of the discipline of economics.

REFERENCES

Culyer, A.J. (1981) 'Health, economics and health economics'. In J. Van Der Gaag and M. Perlman (eds), *Health, economics and health economics*. North Holland, Amsterdam.
────── (1985) *Economics*. Basil Blackwell, Oxford.
Dixon, M. and de Metz, A. (1982) 'Management development for Chief Officers in the NHS: report of a survey'. *King's Fund Project Paper no. 35*, King Edward's Hospital Fund for London.
Drummond, M.F. and Mooney, G.H. (1982 and 1983) 'Essentials of health economics'. (series). *British Medical Journal, 285*, 949–50, 1024–5,

1101–2, 1191–2, 1263–4, 1329–31, 1405–6, 1485–6, 1561–3, 1638–9, 1727–8 and *286*, 40–1.

Evans, R. (1984) *Strained mercy: the economics of Canadian health care*. Butterworths, Toronto.

General Medical Council (Education Committee) (1980) *Recommendations on basic medical education*. GMC, London.

Hersh-Cochran, M.S. (1986) *Survey on education and training programmes in health economics*. World Health Organization (Europe), Copenhagen.

Hiatt, H.H. (1981) 'Training physicians in health policy and management'. In Z. Bankowski and J. Corvera Bernardelli (eds), *Medical ethics and medical education*. WHO (for Council of International Organisations of Medical Sciences), Geneva.

Jennett, B. (1984) 'Economic Appraisal'. *British Medical Journal, 288*, 1781–2.

Knox, E.G. (ed.) (1979) *Epidemiology in health care planning*. Handbook sponsored by the International Epidemiological Association and the World Health Organization, Oxford University Press, Oxford.

Mooney, G.H. (1986) *Economics, medicine and health care*. Wheatsheaf, Sussex.

Spoor, C., Mooney, G. and Maynard, A. (1986) 'Teaching health economics'. *British Medical Journal, 292*, (22 March) p. 785.

Thwaites, B. (Chairman) (1977) 'The education and training of senior managers in the National Health Service — a contribution to debate'. *Report of a King's Fund Working Party*, King Edward's Hospital Fund for London.

University of Aberdeen (Health Economics Research Unit) (1986) *Health Economics Correspondence Course* (Course Brochure). HERU, Aberdeen.

University of York (Centre for Health Economics) (1985) *Health Economics at York*. CHE, York.

Williams, A. (1979) 'One economist's view of social medicine'. *Epidemiology and Community Health, 33*, 3–7.

Part Three

The Measurement of Benefits

13

Changing Patterns of Disease

Nicholas Wells

The simplicity of the title of this chapter belies the immense complexities that surround the very concept of disease as well as the difficulties that beset attempts to forecast developments over specified periods of time. On one level, changes in the patterns of disease may simply derive from increases or reductions in the occurrence of known illnesses. But on a more complicated plane, such changes may reflect factors concerned with the dynamics of disease definition rather than genuine shifts in incidence. Thus rising public expectations regarding health have served to redesignate as episodes of illness warranting medical attention many of those instances of minor and short-lived discomfort that were previously tolerated as an unremarkable part of everyday existence. In 1978/9, nearly 23 million days of certified incapacity for work (6.2 per cent of the total) were attributed to sprains, strains, nervousness, debility or headache. This figure was five times that recorded in 1954/5 when these diagnoses collectively accounted for 1.7 per cent of total absence.

Elucidation of the hazards to health associated with certain conditions and action taken to detect otherwise healthy members of the population thereby at risk also lead to changes in the apparent volume of 'disease'. In this context mild to moderate hypertension provides a contemporary example whilst raised cholesterol levels may become the subject of more rigorous investigation in the years ahead. Similarly, the development of new treatments may serve to uncover or reveal more overtly certain forms of ill health in the community. The anti-depressants may be regarded as exemplars of this observation. In the foreseeable future, common baldness (androgenetic alopecia) might even come to be perceived as a treatable 'illness' should current research lead to the listing of hair

157

restoration as a new induction for minoxidil, a medicine currently employed to lower blood pressure.

Disease patterns are also subject to change as a result of the accumulation of understanding about the mechanisms underlying pathological events and the clinical sequelae with which they are associated. New definitions are one consequence of such progress. Thus Reye's syndrome only became recognised as such in the early 1960s (Reye, Morgan and Baral, 1963) and before that time affected individuals would have appeared in morbidity and mortality records according to the predominant clinical features, encephalopathy and liver enlargement. In similar vein, the term 'sudden infant death syndrome' only entered the language of official statistics in 1971 and, following a recent paper in the *British Medical Journal*, the next few years could see an increase in the incidence of 'Lyme disease' and a corresponding reduction in the number of cases of unexplained skin rash, headache and arthritis seen in children (Williams, Rolles and White, 1986).

The foregoing indicates that many factors underlie changing patterns of disease although the analysis clearly does not pretend in any sense to comprehensiveness. Reference has not been made, for example, to the dissent that surrounds the application of the term 'disease' to certain conditions, such as schizophrenia or alcoholism. The observations do, nevertheless, highlight the immense complexities of investigating changes in the patterns of disease. Given too that an examination of the latter requires attention to be paid to the distribution of ill health within the community according to variables such as age, sex and social class, it is clear that a full analysis is beyond the scope of this paper. Instead it limits itself to the more modest target of identifying the principal factors that will influence disease patterns over the next 25 years and this objective is pursued following a brief review of the key developments that have taken place over the last quarter of a century.

ECONOMIC, SOCIAL AND HEALTH GAINS

The 25 years since OHE was first established have witnessed substantial material gains for the *average* person in the UK (Table 13.1). Remuneration levels have out-paced retail price inflation. Consequently, individuals have been left with a surplus of income after basic requirements such as housing and food[1] have been satisfied and this has been spent on an ever-expanding range of consumer items. In the context of accommodation, there have been substantial improvements in the quality of housing since the early 1960s and the proportion of dwellings that are owner-occupied has risen by approaching 50 per cent. And, at the same time, people have acquired more leisure time in which to enjoy their increasing wealth. For those in employment (the proportion of the population of working age experiencing unemployment today is 10 times greater than in 1961) the length of working day — which is being spent by an increasing proportion of the work force in service rather than manufacturing-based occupations — has steadily declined whilst paid holiday entitlement has doubled.

Substantial change has also occurred from what might very loosely be termed a social perspective. The measurement of social class poses many difficulties but the indications are that upward social mobility has been maintained throughout the period under review (Tables 13.2 and 13.3). For example, in 1972 16 per cent of men of working class origin had found their way into the middle class; by 1983 the percentage had risen to 23.6. Also in 1972, over 60 per cent of individuals of working class parentage were themselves in working class jobs but this proportion had fallen to 52.6 per cent by 1983. Part of the explanation for these trends lies in the increasing level of educational attainment: in 1984, 70 per cent of the population in the 25–29 age group held an educational qualification, compared with only 39 per cent among those aged 50–59 years.

Elsewhere in the spectrum of social change, there have been significant changes in household composition. Average household size has fallen from over three persons in 1961 to around two and a half in 1984. Underlying this trend has been a doubling of the proportion of single person households to 25 per cent of today's total. Consequently 10 per cent of the population now live alone compared with only four per cent in 1961. This development reflects a combination of factors including the increasing frequency of marriage dissolution — decrees absolute granted in 1984 were nearly six times the 1961 total — and the growing numbers of people surviving into old age as widows and widowers. The elderly have in fact come to account for an ever greater proportion of the population. Table 13.4 shows that between 1961 and 1984, the numbers of people aged 65 or over increased by 35 per cent and their share of the population rose by 26 per cent.

Alongside these trends in single person households, the proportion of people living in one-parent families with dependent children

159

Table 13.1: Economic and social change in Britain, 1961–84

	1961		1984	
Average weekly earnings Males	£15.35		£152.70	
of manual workers Females	£7.75		£93.50	
Inflation: purchasing power equivalents	£1.00		£6.90	
	14p		£1.00	
Consumer durables: % of households possessing				
Washing machine	64	(1971)	79	
Refrigerator	69	(1971)	94	
Television	91	(1971)	97	
Telephone	38	(1971)	78	
Video	–		25	
Per cent of households with regular use of a car	31		61	
Housing: stock of dwellings	16.4m		21.7m	
: % owner occupied	43		61	
: % of households entirely without				
fixed bath	22.4	(1966)	1.9	(1981)
internal WC	18.4	(1971)	2.7	(1981)
with central heating	34		66	
Unemployment: numbers	292,000		3,271,000	(mid 1985 UK)
as % of workforce	1.3		13.5	(mid 1985 UK)
Work: normal basic hours for full time manual				
males	42.1		39.1	(UK)
Service industries: employees	10,398,000		13,691,000	(UK)
as % of employees in employment	46		64	(UK)

	(1966)	
Holidays: basic entitlement with pay for full time manual employees	97 per cent allowed 2 weeks	95 per cent allowed four weeks or more
Number of holidays (i.e. 4 nights or more away from home) taken by UK residents	36 million, of which 15 per cent abroad	50 million, of which 32 per cent abroad
Households: average size	3.09	2.59
: % one person	12	25
Divorce: decree absolute granted estimated numbers of divorced people not remarried	27,000	157,000
	285,000	1,811,000
Illegitimate births: numbers	48,000	110,000
as % of total live births	6	17 (England and Wales)

Sources: *Social trends* and *Annual abstract of statistics* (HMSO).

Table 13.2: Distribution of the economically active population by occupational category, in 1951, 1961 and 1971 in Britain (percentages by column)

Standardised Census occupational category	1951 Males	1951 Females	1961 Males	1961 Females	1971 Males	1971 Females
Self-employed and higher-grade salaried professionals	2.8	1.0	4.5	1.1	16.1	1.4
Employers and proprietors	5.7	3.2	4.8	3.0	5.2	2.9
Administrators and managers	6.8	2.7	7.5	2.6	9.9	3.3
Lower-grade salaried professionals and technicians	3.0	7.9	4.0	9.2	5.5	10.8
Inspectors, supervisors and foremen	3.3	1.1	3.8	0.9	4.5	1.2
Clerical workers	6.0	20.3	6.5	25.5	6.1	28.0
Sales personnel and shop assistants	4.0	9.6	3.9	10.0	3.9	9.4
Skilled manual workers (inc. self-employed artisans)	30.3	12.7	32.3	10.8	29.4	9.3
Semi-skilled manual workers	24.3	33.6	22.8	30.9	21.2	27.3
Unskilled manual workers	13.8	7.9	9.9	6.0	8.2	6.4
Total active population (thousands)	15,584	6,903	15,992	7,649	15,609	8,762

Source: Halsey, 1986.

Table 13.3: Class distribution of respondents by class of father, 1972 and (1983) inquiries

Father's class	Respondent's class (percentages by row)		
	Middle class	Lower-middle	Working class
Middle class	57.7 (62.0)	23.3 (22.2)	19.1 (15.8)
Lower-middle	31.2 (34.2)	31.9 (34.3)	37.0 (31.5)
Working class	16.0 (23.6)	23.7 (23.8)	61.2 (52.6)

Source: Halsey, 1986.

Table 13.4: The UK population in 1961 and 1984

Age group	1961	Per cent of total	1984	Per cent of total
0–14	12.336	23.4	10.997	19.5
15–44	20.783	39.4	24.498	43.4
45–64	13.399	25.4	12.606	22.3
65+	6.190	11.7	8.387	14.8
	52.708	100	56.488	100

Source: *Annual abstract of statistics* (HMSO).

has doubled since 1961 to reach 5 per cent in 1983. This development reflects the rising divorce rate noted above, the increasing incidence of illegitimate births — the latter now account for 17 per cent of all live births, three times the proportion of 1961 — and fewer illegitimate children being put forward for adoption.

The perhaps surprisingly extensive changes in British society that have taken place in the relatively short period of time since the start of the 1960s have played varying roles in the equally profound shifts in the nation's health. Table 13.5 presents male and female mortality rates in 1962 and 1984 in the UK. In the absence of the overall reductions indicated, it may be estimated that in 1984 there would have been 30,000 more deaths than were actually recorded. In particular, the period saw a continuation of the successful battle against infectious diseases — the mortality rate for this group of causes fell by almost 60 per cent between 1962 and 1984.[2]

Age specific data show that the most substantial reductions in death rates occurred among the younger groups (Table 13.5). In particular, there was a notable improvement in infant mortality. Figure 13.1 reveals that deaths under one year of age fell from 22.4 per 1,000 live births in 1962 to 9.6 per 1,000 in 1984. Without this 57 per cent improvement the toll of infant mortality in 1984 would

163

Table 13.5: UK mortality rates per 1,000 population

	Males		Females	
Age group	1962	1984	1962	1984
0–4	6.4	2.6	4.9	2.0
5–9	0.5	0.3	0.3	0.2
10–14	0.4	0.3	0.3	0.2
15–19	0.9	0.7	0.4	0.3
20–24	1.1	0.9	0.5	0.3
25–34	1.1	0.9	0.8	0.5
35–44	2.5	1.7	1.8	1.2
45–54	7.4	5.7	4.5	3.5
55–64	22.5	17.5	11.0	9.7
65–74	54.8	44.9	30.7	24.3
75–84	124.2	100.9	87.2	62.6
85+	265.5	212.8	226.4	170.2
All ages	12.6	11.7	11.3	11,2

Source: *Annual abstract of statistics* (HMSO).

have been greater by 180 deaths every week. Against this background, life expectancy at birth in the UK has risen for males from 67.9 years in 1961 to 71.1 years in 1981–3. For females the corresponding extension was from 73.8 to 77 years.

Focusing on morbidity, there have been numerous pharmaceutical and surgical advances that have yielded improvements in the quality of life for patients suffering from a wide range of diseases. Effective new medicines based on a clearer understanding of the role of chemicals and receptors within various physiological systems have become available for the treatment of asthma, angina, Parkinson's disease and peptic ulceration. Other pharmaceutical innovations since the early 1960s include oral contraceptives, antiviral medicines, improved psychotropic preparations and powerful immunosuppressant agents. The latter have played a key part in the progress that has been achieved in heart transplanation. By the end of 1984 a total of 277 heart transplants had been undertaken at Papworth and Harefield hospitals since the start of the programme in 1979. Kidney transplantation, too, only became a realistic alternative to dialysis in 1960 when the first immunosuppressive drug became available and in 1985 almost 1,500 patients received a transplant. Coronary artery bypass grafts, cardiac pacemakers, total hip replacements (more than 25,000 were carried out in England alone in 1984) and corneal transplants are further examples of surgical interventions that have effectively 'taken-off' since the early 1960s.

Figure 13.1: Infant mortality in the UK 1962–84, rates per 1,000 live births

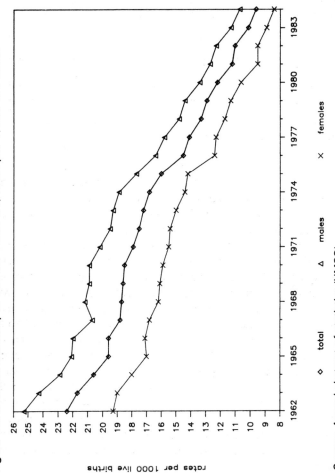

Source: *Annual abstract of statistics* (HMSO).

The period has of course also witnessed a number of trends that counterbalance the positive developments described above. Senile dementia, for example, has emerged as a substantial problem. The prevalence of moderate or severe dementia among those aged 65 years or more has been estimated at between 6 and 7 per cent. Consequently, the number of affected individuals in the UK has risen more than 35 per cent between 1961 and 1984 to reach almost 560,000 in the latter year.

Coronary heart disease (CHD) has risen to prominence as a major cause of (avoidable) ill health in contemporary society. In 1961, CHD was responsible for 26,912 deaths between the ages of 35 and 64 years in Britain. This was equivalent to a rate of 2.78 per 1,000 population. In 1984 this number had increased to 29,051 or 3.00 per 1,000 population. Although neither of the measures has increased substantially, the reduction in mortality from other causes has meant that the proportion of deaths attributable to CHD in this age group has risen almost 40 per cent over the period to reach 38 per cent in 1984.

Other significant 'negative' developments since the early 1960s include the rising prevalence of attempted suicide (or perhaps more accurately, deliberate self harm) and of drug and alcohol abuse.

Accurate data on the first of these are not available but there is general agreement that the annual number of episodes rose sharply during the 1970s to reach 100,000 per annum by the end of the decade. With regard to alcohol abuse there has been a steady increase in *per capita* consumption in the UK among people aged 15 and over from 5.2 litres in 1960 to 8.9 litres in 1984. Linked with this trend has been a rise in admissions to mental illness hospitals and units with a diagnosis of alcohol misuse from 24.8 per 100,000 population in 1973 to 36.7 in 1983 and a trebling of the death rate for alcohol related liver disease to 17.9 per million over the same period. As in the case of deliberate self harm, figures relating to the occurrence of drug abuse are inadequate but one estimate suggests that more than 60,000 people regularly misuse drugs and that the most frequently involved substance is heroin (Braine, 1986). Underlying trends in this area are a source of considerable concern: in the UK the number of new addicts to narcotic drugs notified to the Home Office totalled 5,415 in 1984, 5.5 times the 1976 total.

PREDICTING THE FUTURE

It is unlikely that many of the wide-ranging developments described above would have been foreseen with much, if any, accuracy at the outset of the 1960s. Equally, there can be little certainty concerning the patterns that might unfold over the next 25 years. Morbidity and mortality trends are no less subject to the unexpected than anything else. Few would claim to have predicted the epidemic of asthma deaths among young people during the 1960s or the sharp decline in pertussis vaccine acceptance rates in the 1970s which heralded the recrudescence of whooping cough epidemics on a scale that had not been experienced since 1957, when vaccination was recommended on a national scale.

A more recent and extremely forceful reminder of the hazards of forecasting disease patterns is of course provided by acquired immune deficiency syndrome (AIDS). AIDS is a new and highly lethal disease in man. It first emerged at the start of the 1980s in the United States and the number of cases has grown at an alarming pace: the 7,691 cases and 3,661 deaths recorded by the end of 1984 had more than doubled to 16,500 and 8,500 respectively just 12 months later. Similar rates of progression have been reported in the UK and the Chief Medical Officer of the Department of Health and Social Security has stated that 'controlling the spread of infection must be regarded as an issue of prime importance to the future of the nation' (Acheson, 1986).

In addition to the ever present risk of the unexpected event, forecasting is inhibited by the inevitable absence of measures suitable for tracking over time and projecting into the future. In many instances the guides that are available cover only a limited area of interest and reflect the provision of treatment rather than the volume of ill health in the community. The latest survey of morbidity in general practice, for example, relates to 1981/2 and indicates that 65 per cent of males and 77 per cent of females consult their family doctor at least once during the course of any given year. Table 13.6 shows that these proportions were greater than those found in the 1971/2 survey by 5.2 per cent and 9.2 per cent respectively. Indeed, all age groups with the exception of males aged 15–24 years experienced an increase in patients' consulting rates over the decade. Together with the findings of the first in this series of surveys, which was carried out in the 1950s, data could theoretically be projected forward to provide some measure of future levels of ill health.

167

Table 13.6: Patients consulting in general practice, rates per 1,000 persons at risk

Age group	Males 1971/2	Males 1981/2	Females 1971/2	Females 1981/2
0–4	891.5	991.3	874.9	977.5
5–14	611.9	661.3	616.1	676.4
15–24	584.8	582.6	755.8	819.4
25–44	574.6	579.4	726.1	766.9
45–64	605.5	630.9	665.0	716.7
65–74	644.5	720.7	660.7	753.0
75+	662.5	777.1	662.1	795.0
All ages	622.3	652.2	700.0	765.8

Source: OPCS Monitor MB5 86/1.

However, apart from the inaccuracies inherent in prediction based on just three data points, each separated by an interval of a decade or more, this approach is subject to a number of other limitations. It is, for example, axiomatic that data presented at a global level do not reveal important temporal changes in the relative significance of consultations for minor discomforts, major illness and for preventive medicine. In addition, the figures do not reflect the true level of ill health in the community because they exclude episodes of illness which individuals either ignore, treat themselves or for which help is obtained from other sources such as practitioners of alternative medicine or hospital clinics (not infrequently, in cases of what some commentators regard as the 'very stuff' of general practice, such as the long term management of diabetes or hypertension). General practice consultation data also fail to take account of the services supplied by members of the primary health care team other than the doctor. In this context, the General Household Survey found that 7 per cent of individuals aged 65 years or more received care from either a district nurse or health visitor in the month preceding interview in 1983.

Data based on hospital inpatient treatment are generally biased towards the more serious end of the spectrum of ill health and are consequently yet more limited as guides of the prevalence of disease. Furthermore, changes in hospital admissions reflect the interaction of a mix of factors including resource availability, the influence of technological advance on the boundaries of (and responsibility for) treatable illness and new approaches to care which may raise or lower the propensity to admit to hospital. Such considerations, rather than marked shifts in the occurrence of disease, probably

Figure 13.2: Hospital discharges in England 1979–84, numbers and rates per 1,000 population

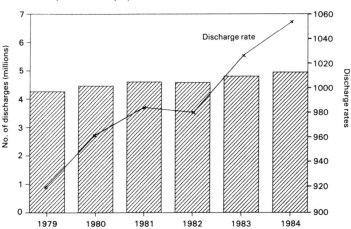

Source: OPCS Monitor MB4 86/1.

account for much of the 15 per cent increase in the hospital discharge rate between 1979 and 1984 shown in Figure 13.2. It might also be added that the usefulness of inpatient data in isolation is becoming yet more limited with the continuing increase in the scope for day care treatment and investigation. In 1983, day cases accounted for 14 per cent of the total hospital treated cases in England and 23 per cent of all operations performed. In 1979 the corresponding proportions were 12 per cent and 20 per cent respectively.

Figures reflecting service usage therefore provide only limited information about changing morbidity patterns within the population. An alternative approach might be to focus instead on mortality data. Figure 13.3 compares national mortality profiles for 1951 and 1983 and indicates in broad terms that among younger persons the infectious diseases have been replaced by accidents as the principal cause of death whilst the cancers and circulatory diseases have come to dominate middle age mortality patterns. Table 13.7 indicates in more detail the contemporary situation for England and, in a sense, thereby identifies the targets for the next 25 years.

As with the service usage data, it is theoretically possible to extrapolate from the trends shown in Figure 13.3 to obtain a broad outline of the mortality patterns that might prevail a decade or so into the next century. But once again questions concerning the nature of

169

Figure 13.3: Selected causes of death by age and sex, Britain*, 1951 and 1983

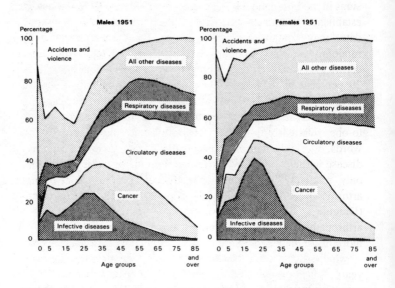

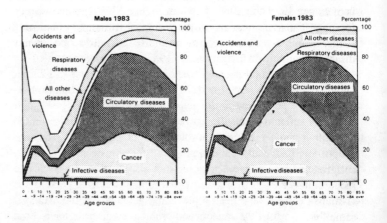

*1983 figures are for the UK.
Source: *Social trends* (HMSO).

the data themselves generate doubts about the worth of conducting such exercises. In addition to problems arising from periodic revisions in the International Classification of Disease (ICD), it has been established that death certificates, the basis of national mortality data, may contain significant errors. One recent study of 272 randomly selected autopsy reports and corresponding death certificates identified disagreements on such an extensive scale that 29 per cent of the deaths had to be reclassified into a new ICD category (Kircher, Nelson and Burdo, 1985).

However, the principal shortcoming lies in the absence of a one-to-one relationship between mortality and morbidity. In other words, mortality data may be an inadequate guide to patterns of disease in the community because certain major causes of disability only relatively infrequently directly cause death. For example, arthritis affects 41 per cent of the population aged 65 years or more (Dreghorn, Roughneen, Graham and Hamblen, 1986) yet all arthropathies and related disorders account for only 0.6 per cent of mortality at these ages. Similarly, the significance of senile dementia — which affects more than half a million people over the age of 65 years — is not reflected in the total of 7,260 deaths attributed to the condition in 1984 (figures for England and Wales). In addition there is of course the obvious point that whilst mortality data might appear to suggest that individuals suffer from one principal condition in reality many people experience contemporaneously two or more disabling conditions for substantial periods of their lives.

An alternative approach to investigating patterns of disease which avoids the problems inherent in service usage and mortality data is to conduct surveys among the population. This methods is adopted by the General Household Survey which has been conducted annually since the early 1970s. Figures 13.4 and 13.5 show the proportion of individuals indicating in the 1983 survey that they had suffered from restricted activity in the 14 days preceding interview (acute illness). For males the responses appear to generate a shallow U-shaped curve whilst for females reporting rates remain within the same broad limits throughout the age spectrum. In contrast the patterns for long-standing illness, and for long-standing illness that limits activity, demonstrate a steady increase with age for both sexes.

Data from the General Household Survey over the period 1972–83 (Figure 13.6) reveal increases in self-reported chronic ill health from 20 to 31 per cent for males and from 21 to 33 per cent for females. The prevalence of long-standing illness therefore appears

171

Table 13.7: Five main causes at different ages (and percentages of all causes of deaths) England, 1984

A

RANK	All ages Males %	All ages Females %	1–14 Males %	1–14 Females %	15–34 Males %	15–34 Females %	35–54 Males %	35–54 Females %	55–74 Males %	55–74 Females %	75 and over Males %	75 and over Females %
1	Ischaemic heart disease 31	Ischaemic heart disease 24	Road vehicle accidents 21	Road vehicle accidents 16	Road vehicle accidents 29	Road vehicle accidents 15	Ischaemic heart disease 35	M.N. of bone connective tissue, skin and breast 21	Ischaemic heart disease 37	Ischaemic heart disease 26	Ischaemic heart disease 28	Ischaemic heart disease 25
2	M.N. of respiratory and intra-thoracic organs 10	Cerebro-vascular disease 16	Other causes of injury and poisoning 19	Congenital anomalies 15	Other cause of injury and poisoning 18	Other causes of injury and poisoning 11	M.N. of digestive organs and peritoneum 9	M.N. of genito-urinary organs 11	M.N. of respiratory and intra-thoracic organs 12	Cerebro-vascular disease 11	Cerebro-vascular disease 13	Cerebro-vascular disease 19
3	Cerebro-vascular disease 10	Other diseases of the circulatory system 10	Congenital anomalies 13	Other causes of injury and poisoning 13	Suicide and self-inflicted injury 13	M.N. of bone connective tissue, skin and breast 9	M.N. of respiratory and intra-thoracic organs 9	Ischaemic heart disease 10	M.N. of digestive organs and peritoneum 9	M.N. of digestive organs and peritoneum 9	Other diseases of the circulatory system 9	Other diseases of the circulatory system 13
4	M.N. of digestive organs and peritoneum 8	M.N. of digestive organs and peritoneum 7	Diseases of the nervous system and sense organs 9	Diseases of the nervous system and sense organs 10	Diseases of the nervous system and sense organs 5	Suicide and self-inflicted injury 7	Suicide and self-inflicted injury 5	M.N. of digestive organs and peritoneum 8	Cerebro-vascular disease 8	M.N. of bone connective tissue, skin and breast 8	Chronic obstructive pulmonary disease and allied conditions 8	Pneumonia 8

	Other diseases of the circulatory system	Pneumonia	M.N.* of lymphatic and haemato-poietic tissue	M.N. of lymphatic and haemato-poietic tissue	M.N. of lymphatic and haemato-poietic tissue	Diseases of nervous system and sense organs	Cerebro-vascular disease	Cerebro-vascular disease	Chronic obstructive pulmonary disease and allied conditions	M.N. of respiratory and intra-thoracic organs	M.N. of respiratory and intra-thoracic organs	M.N. of respiratory and intra-thoracic organs
	7	5	8	6	5	7	5	6	6	7	7	6
Remainder 34	38		30	40	30	51	37	44	28	39	35	29
All causes of death	264,182	267,182	1,332	916	5,792	2,656	19,181	12,091	121,836	80,006	112,802	169,030
	100	100	100	100	100	100	100	100	100	100	100	100

5

Source: On the state of the public health for the year 1984 (HMSO).
Note: M.N. = malignant neoplasm.

Figure 13.4: Proportion of males reporting acute, long standing and limiting long standing ill health in 1983

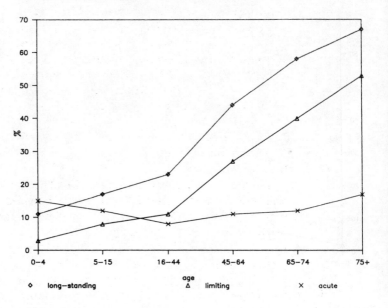

Source: *General household survey.*

to have increased by about 50 per cent for both sexes in the space of slightly more than a decade. If this trend continues then prevalence could rise to 58 per cent and 65 per cent for males and females respectively by 2012.

The simple regressions against time which underlie these estimates have of course to be treated with caution. The hazards of the approach may be illustrated in the context of AIDS. On the basis of the increase in the number of cases seen up to the end of 1984, simple extrapolations suggest that the annual number of new AIDS cases will equate with the size of the entire UK population at the turn of the century! In fact the data contained in Figure 13.6 indicate that the steady increase in self-reported chronic ill health witnessed in the 1970s came to a halt at the start of the 1980s. Prevalence rates then levelled out for a short time only to resume an upward trend in 1983. Future developments are uncertain.

Equally unclear are the factors underlying the rising prevalence

Figure 13.5: Proportion of females reporting acute, long standing and limiting long standing ill health in 1983

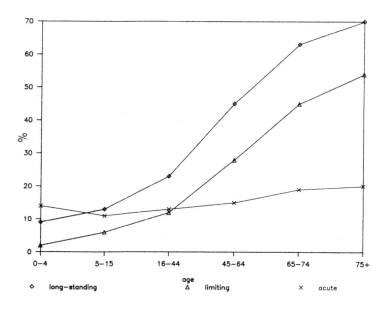

Source: *General household survey.*

Figure 13.6: Proportion of males and females in Britain reporting long standing illness, 1972–83

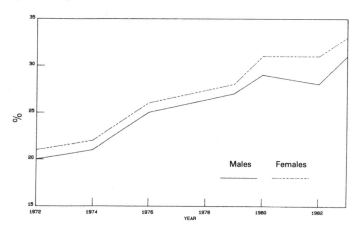

Source: *General household survey.*

175

of chronic ill health. They are not solely a function of the ageing of the population since substantial increases in prevalence have occurred among all age groups. It seems likely that a combination of factors must be involved and these include ever-increasing expectations on the part of the public regarding acceptable levels of health and perhaps changes in the prevalence and duration of chronic sickness. Given this degree of uncertainty, it might be suggested that the time is ripe for a new survey of impairment and handicap in Britain. The data flowing from the General Household Survey certainly appear to suggest that the findings of Harris' original survey of this area in the late 1960s must now be rather dated.

FUTURE INFLUENCES ON DISEASE PATTERNS

The foregoing has made clear that forecasts of the future — especially as far ahead as 25 years — are likely to be subject to considerable error. It is nevertheless possible to highlight a number of elements that will clearly be relevant to changes in the patterns of disease over the next quarter century.

The first of these factors is the continuing process of demographic transition. The population of the UK is projected to increase between 1984 and 2013 by 2.9 per cent to reach 58.12 million. Within this total, persons aged 65 and over will increase by 13 per cent from 8.39 million to 9.50 million. And within this subgroup, the old elderly, that is people over 75 years will increase 16 per cent from 3.54 million in 1984 to 4.11 million in 2013. The elderly as a whole will therefore increase their representation within the total population from 14.8 per cent in 1984 to 16.3 per cent in 2013. These trends, in conjunction with the rising prevalence of chronic ill health in old age, have clear implications for illness patterns over the next 25 years although, as Figure 13.7 shows, the 'burden' linked to the ageing population will not maintain steady upward growth throughout the entire period.

Technological advance, that is, increasingly accurate understanding of the mechanisms underpinning disease processes and the translation of such progress into effective means of prevention or therapeutic intervention, could obviously have a major impact on future patterns of disease. The present time appears to be one of immense excitement in research and potential exists for advance on a broad range of disease fronts. This is particularly the case in 'genetic illness' which has become increasingly significant with the

Figure 13.7: The elderly in the UK population 1984–2013

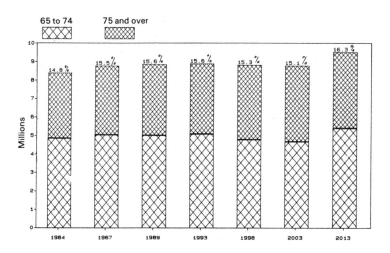

Note: Percentage shown at the top of each stack is the poportion of the total population accounted for by the over 65s as a whole.
Source: *Annual abstract of statistics* (HMSO).

decline of infectious disease. According to McKusick's *Mendelian inheritance in man*, some 3,000 human diseases arising from genetic defects have been identified to date. It is estimated that between 3 and 10 babies out of every 1,000 are born with a serious single gene disorder such as haemophilia or cystic fibrosis. Chromosomal abnormalities, such as that responsible for Down's syndrome, are even more common affecting about 6 per 1,000 births. In addition to this toll, genetic factors may contribute to some congenital malformations and cases of mental retardation,[3] as well as to some common adult disorders such as diabetes, schizophrenia and coronary heart disease (Weatherall, 1984). Genes with important functions in the regulation of cell division and growth — the oncogenes — also appear to be involved in different stages of neoplastic transformation.

At the present time, the cause of many genetic diseases and the chromosomal location of the genes involved are unknown. However, progress in biotechnology has yielded genetic probes which are enabling scientists to get closer to the genetic defects underlying

177

such diseases at Huntington's chorea, muscular dystrophy, poly-cystic kidney disease and cystic fibrosis. Continuing advance in this area could have a major impact on future disease patterns. This might be effected via, for example, a considerably extended use of pre-natal screening, based on analyses of DNA obtained by chorion villus sampling or amniocentesis, and subsequent pregnancy termination where considered desirable. Alternatively, screening at this stage or post-natally might facilitate identification of those with a genetic predisposition to disorders such as coronary artery disease and thus open the way for potentially more effective preventive strategies. A further possibility lies in the development of gene therapy. The latter might involve taking cells from a 'genetically compromised' person, isolating and removing the defective gene sequence and inserting the correct one. If these cells can then be reintroduced to the patient so that they both multiply and express the corrected gene, then the disease may be ameliorated or even cured (Hodgkin and Yoxen, 1985).

Against this background, Weatherall (1986) has commented that 'the next few years will see a major change in emphasis in medical research from the "whole patient" to the cellular and molecular pathology of disease processes. This should help to dissect the complex interactions of genotype and environment which underlie many of the common killing diseases of western societies'.

Recombinant DNA technology will also have important clinical applications outside genetics. To date it has been employed to produce a number of physiologically active polypeptides and examples of those that already have direct therapeutic uses include insulin, factor VIII and interferon. In addition, endorphins, the opiate like substances found in brain tissue, have been cloned and work is now in progress to develop compounds that will exploit and perhaps amplify the analgesic and mood-altering characteristics of endorphins. New knowledge should generate further novel therapeutic agents and vaccines — recombinant technology offers an efficient method of obtaining large amounts of uncontaminated antigen for a range of diseases including perhaps AIDS, herpes and dental caries (Hodgkin and Yoxen, 1985).

The prospects for future progress in the effective treatment of viruses are becoming brighter with increasing understanding of the molecular events underlying viral replication. Discoveries relating to the enzymes that are crucial to certain viruses for the synthesis of their own nuclear material as well as progress in the sequencing of the genetic structure of human viruses could, in the next decade

Table 13.8: Susceptibility of viruses to chemotherapy

	Available	Under investigation	Unavailable
DNA viruses	Herpes simplex Varicella zoster Variola, vaccinia	Hepatitis B Cytomegalovirus	Parvoviruses Papovaviruses Adenoviruses Epstein-Barr virus
RNA viruses	Influenza A	Influenza B Respiratory syncytial virus Rhinoviruses HTLV-III	Enteroviruses Reoviruses Togaviruses Arenaviruses Coronaviruses Bunyaviruses Rhabdoviruses Lentiviruses

Source: Collier, 1986.

or so, radically alter the contemporary therapeutic situation described in Table 13.8.

Monoclonal antibodies constitute another product with major significance for diagnosis and treatment to emerge from molecular biological research. These agents should become increasingly useful in detecting tumour cells and have potential for the imaging of lesions in deep tissues or the localisation of tumours in small foci inaccessible to other diagnostic tests. However Dick (1985) suggests that 'the greatest potential benefit is likely to be derived from the use of monoclonal antibodies as carriers of drugs or toxins for the efficient localisation of cytotoxic treatments'. In addition to carrying conventional cytotoxic agents such as methotrexate and adriamycin, the use of radioisotope — labelled monoclonal antibodies — is also being studied in the context of cancer therapy (Baldwin and Byers, 1986).

Equally rapid progress is also being achieved in other areas of medical science — for example, in unravelling the biochemistry of the brain. The earlier picture of nerve impulse transmission under the regulation of chemical messengers such as L-glutamate, acetylcholine and dopamine is now recognised to be too simplistic following the discovery of a new class of modulatory chemical signals in the brain, the neuropeptides. At the present time 40 of these substances have been identified. Neuropeptide and monoamine signalling is immensely complex but with further clarification new approaches to the treatment of mental and neurological illness

179

should become available as ways of manipulating the chemistry of the brain are discovered (Iversen, 1985).

It is not possible to predict when the fruits of research in these and other areas will become available in the form of effective therapy. In this regard it is instructive to return to molecular biology. DNA was established as a self-replicating double helix in the 1950s. But this and associated discoveries had little impact on the clinical world and in the early 1970s Burnet (1973) wrote 'I cannot avoid the conclusion that we have reached the stage in 1971 when little further advance can be expected from laboratory science in the handling of the intrinsic types of disability and disease'. Subsequently, there has been a new wave of advance and, according to Weatherall (1986), 'clinical scientists have started to see the extraordinary potential of what molecular biology has on offer'.

Yet a more fundamental issue than the timing of the arrival of the benefits of technological progress revolves around the question of whether sufficient resources will be available in the first instance to finance the necessary research initiatives. Elsewhere (Wells, 1986) it has been pointed out that public funds for medical research have been severely constrained in recent times and that charitable bodies are assuming an increasing responsibility for sustaining the UK's effort in this field. Although the rapid take-off of this compensatory source of funds is clearly to be welcomed, there is some anxiety that charitable finance is not generally channelled — at least at present — towards the long term fundamental areas of investigation that could well underpin the major therapeutic breakthroughs of the future.

Remaining with issues of finance, a third factor that will have a bearing on changes in the future pattern of disease is the support made available to the health services. The relationship between the latter and the health of the community is extremely complex and the subject of considerable, not to say at times unhelpfully polarised, debate. In a recent paper from Finland, however, it was calculated that the health services accounted for 50 per cent of the total decline in mortality from amenable causes between 1969 and 1981 (Poikolainen and Eskola, 1986). This estimate accords broadly with the conclusions of a study based on mortality in England and Wales over the period 1974–83 (Lakhani, Charlton and Aristidou, 1986).

Against a background of these findings and similar observations in the context of morbidity, the financial difficulties currently being endured by the health service are a source of concern. Shortfalls in the form of long waiting lists (at the end of 1984 there were two patients awaiting admission to an NHS hospital for each occupied bed) and those of a less tangible nature related to the quality of care are the product of a growing imbalance between the demand for and supply of health care resources. Looking to the future, it seems certain that the pressures driving the demand side of the equation — rising health expectations, technological advance and the ageing population — will continue to intensify. Consequently, unless appropriate supply-side solutions are forthcoming, the nation's capacity to deliver desired levels of effective health care will diminish.

In this respect, a reordering of public spending priorities — defence accounted for 13.3 per cent of government expenditure in 1984 and as such received £200 million more than the NHS — is widely seen as a key requirement. But political uncertainties, in conjunction with the economic realities imposed by the nation's prosperity, also dictate that full value must be gained from the resources available to the health sector. Considerable attention is therefore being directed towards potentially more efficient means of health care supply in the future. One of the models most frequently discussed in this regard is the Health Maintenance Organisation which has its origins in the United States. Experiments with such approaches to health care, or variants upon them, are to be welcomed. However, as the most recent report to emerge from the Rand Health Insurance Study makes clear (Ware *et al.*, 1986), attention needs to be paid as much to the outputs of potential new systems of delivery as to the organisation of resource inputs if already existing patterns of social inequality in health are not to be further exaggerated.

The fourth factor, or set of factors, that may be expected to influence the picture of disease in the future follows directly on from the last point. There exists a considerable body of evidence concerning the influence of many different social variables on health. The isolation and quantification of these effects is a complex field of analysis and forecasting potential developments adds yet another dimension of difficulty and uncertainty. There is, however, little dispute that unemployment has become, and seems set to remain, a major determinant of health status.

The increasing levels of unemployment — a fourfold rise to 3.2 million between 1975 and 1985 — have generated considerable research interest in the health sequelae of job loss. An analysis of mortality in the period 1971–81 found a 20–30 per cent excess among men who in 1971 had been seeking work and an excess of around 20 per cent for the wives of these men (Moser, Fox, Jones

Figure 13.8: Mortality by social class among males aged 15–65 years, in 1970–72, England and Wales

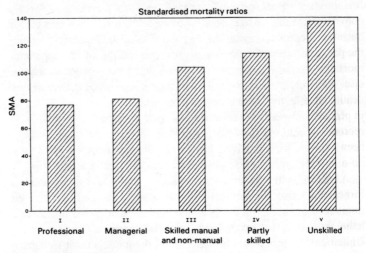

Source: Black, 1980.

and Goldblatt, 1984). Suicide was an especially frequent cause of death and the incidence of attempted suicide has also been shown to be higher among unemployed men than those with jobs — a recent investigation in Oxford found a 12–15-fold difference (Hawton and Rose, 1986). New studies from general practice further indicate that threatened job loss, actual redundancy and forced premature retirement are associated with increased morbidity as measured by increased consultations, episodes of illness and referrals to hospital outpatient clinics (Beale and Nethercott, 1986a, 1986b). Findings such as these clearly demonstrate the need for appropriate employment strategies as the UK enters an era requiring further change in the skills of the workforce and in which the overall demand for labour will probably continue to decline. Failure to construct effective policies will not only serve to increase the extent of physical and mental disorder in absolute terms but, given the higher rates of unemployment among the least skilled members of the community, shortcomings in this respect could also magnify the existing social inequalities in health status indicated in Figure 13.8.

A final factor that will have a major bearing on the future pattern of disease will be the success that is achieved in advancing disease prevention and health promotion. In the 1982 Harveian Oration,

Doll (1983) argued that modifications of personal habits offer the greatest opportunities for disease prevention and he identified in particular smoking and, albeit more speculatively, diet. Universal abandonment of the former habit would reduce mortality from all cancers by one third, almost eliminate chronic obstructive lung disease and the complications of peripheral vascular disease and cut mortality from myocardial infarction by a quarter. The last mentioned, as Table 13.7 indicates, is a major cause of premature mortality.

It is of course encouraging that the prevalence of cigarette smoking has fallen by 31 per cent and 22 per cent among males and females respectively over the period 1972–84. Nevertheless, it may be estimated that cigarettes are still smoked by 14.8 million people in Britain (34 per cent of the population) and that 1.6 million in this group are under 20 years of age. As a result the habit continues to be a major factor in the deaths of 100,000 people each year, one quarter of whom are under 65 years of age (Fowler, 1984).

The elimination of, or very substantial reductions in, cigarette smoking could therefore emerge as the largest single influence on disease patterns over the next 25 years. The extent to which this particular goal and indeed all of the other objectives throughout the entire spectrum of disease prevention and health promotion are realised will depend on a range of factors including resource availability, the enthusiasm of those charged with the responsibility of dispensing 'preventive care', the utilisation of economic and other incentives and, where relevant, suitable legislation. But arguably one of the most important determinants of success in this area will be the extent to which advantage is taken of the opportunities for health education provided by the years spent at school.

CONCLUSION

This paper has resisted the temptation to speculate directly upon the patterns of disease that might prevail a decade or so into the next century. Instead it has made clear that many different and frequently interacting factors will have a bearing on the future health of the nation and that the sum of their effects cannot be predicted so far ahead with any degree of confidence. This does not of course mean that an appropriate 'health target' for the next 25 years cannot be identified. Indeed, *pace* Fries (1980), the objective must be to enable increasing numbers to enjoy the 'ideal average life span' of about 85 years and to compress the experience of chronic morbidity into ever smaller periods of time towards the end of that span. In simple terms, this might be seen to require a two fold strategy: preventive initiatives directed towards the major causes of premature death (such as coronary heart disease) and therapeutic innovation to ameliorate the morbidity from, if not actually eliminate, the chronic diseases of later life.

NOTES

1. Food accounted for almost 25 per cent of consumer expenditure in 1961 compared with less than 15 per cent in 1984.

2. Based on data for England and Wales.

3. In broad terms, genetic disorders along with congenital malformations occur in 2–5 per cent of all live births, account for nearly a third of all paediatric admissions and cause 40–50 per cent of deaths in childhood (Weatherall, 1984).

REFERENCES

Acheson, D. (1986) *On the state of the public health for the year 1984*. HMSO, London.

Baldwin, R.W. and Byers, V.S. (1986) 'Monoclonal antibodies in cancer treatment'. *Lancet, 1*, 603–5.

Beale, N. and Nethercott, S. (1986a) 'Job-loss and health — the influence of old age and previous morbidity'. *J. Roy. Coll. Gen. Pract., 36*, 261–4.

———— and ———— (1986b) 'Job-loss and morbidity in a group of employees nearing retirement age'. *J. Roy. Coll. Gen. Pract., 36*, 265–6.

Black, D. (1980) *Inequalities in health*. DHSS, London.

Braine, B. (1986) *Hansard*, 6 March, col. 561.

Burnet, F.M. (1973) *Dreams, genes and realities*. Penguin Books, Aylesbury.

Collier, L.H. (1986) 'Antiviral drugs'. *Update*, 1 April.

Dick, H.M. (1985) 'Monoclonal antibodies in clinical medicine'. *British Medical Journal, 291*, 762–4.

Doll, R. (1983) 'Prospects for prevention'. *British Medical Journal, 286*, 445–53.

Dreghorn, C.R., Roughneen, P., Graham, J. and Hamblen, D.L. (1986) 'The real cost of joint replacement'. *British Medical Journal, 1*, 1636–7.

Fowler, G. (1984) 'Smoking'. *Update*, 15 March.

Fries, J.F. (1980) 'Aging, natural death, and the compression of morbidity'. *New England Journal of Medicine, 303*, 130–5.

Halsey, A.H. (1986) *Change in British society*, 3rd edn. Oxford University

Press, Oxford.

Harris, A.I., Cox, E. and Smith, R.W. (1971) *Handicapped and impaired in Britain, Part 1*. HMSO, London.

Hawton, K. and Rose, N. (1986) 'Unemployment and attempted suicide among men in Oxford'. *Health Trends, 18*, 29–32.

Hodgkin, P. and Yoxen, E. (1985) 'Biotechnology and general practice. Recombinant DNA, monoclonal antibodies and genetic probes'. *J. Roy. Coll. Gen. Pract., 35*, 484–7.

Iversen, L. (1985) 'Chemicals to think by'. *New Scientist*, 30 May.

Kircher, T., Nelson, J. and Burdo, H. (1985) 'The autopsy as a measure of accuracy of the death certificate'. *New England Journal of Medicine, 313*, 20, 1263–9.

Lakhani, A., Charlton, J. and Aristidou, M. (1986) 'Mortality from causes amenable to health services intervention'. *Lancet, 1*, 1029.

Moser, K.A., Fox, A.J., Jones, D.R. and Goldblatt, P.O. (1986) 'Unemployment and mortality: further evidence from the OPCS Longitudinal Study 1971–81'. *Lancet, 1*, 365–7.

Poikolainen, K. and Eskola, J. (1986) 'The effect of Health Services on mortality: decline in death rates from amenable and non-amenable causes in Finland 1969–81'. *Lancet, 1*, 199–202.

Reye, R.D.K., Morgan, G. and Baral, J. (1963) 'Encephalopathy and fatty degeneration of the viscera: a disease entity in childhood'. *Lancet, 2*, 749–52.

Ware, J.E., Brook, R.H., Rogers, W.H., Keeler, E.B., Davies, A., Sherbourne, C., Goldberg, G.A., Camp, P. and Newhouse, J.P. (1986) 'Comparison of health outcomes at a Health Maintenance Organisation with those of fee-for-service care'. *Lancet, 1*, 1017–22.

Weatherall, D. (1984) 'On the track of genetic disease'. *New Scientist*, 5 April.

—— (1986) 'Molecular biology at the bedside'. *British Medical Journal, 292*, 1505–8.

Wells, N.E.J. (1986) *Crisis in research*. OHE, London.

Williams, D., Rolles, C.J. and White, J.E. (1986) 'Lyme disease in a Hampshire child — medical curiosity or beginning of an epidemic?' *British Medical Journal, 1*, 1560–1.

14

Cost Benefit Analysis in Health Care: Future Directions

Michael Drummond

INTRODUCTION

The term 'cost benefit analysis' is used to describe a family of techniques which all seek to assess alternative projects, programmes or activities from the viewpoint of economic efficiency. The general justification for economic evaluation is that given scarcity of resources tough choices need to be made on how these are deployed. It was recognised in the early 1960s that the health care sector, given its importance in the economies of most developed countries, could not be immune from such evaluation and the first studies began to appear (Weisbrod, 1961; Klarman, 1965).

Much of the early work was exploratory, dealing with issues such as how to measure the benefits of commodities like health care, for which market prices were not readily available (Mishan, 1971). However, the extent of empirical investigation broadened greatly through the 1970s and by the early 1980s there were a number of general methodological texts and critical reviews of published work in the health care field (Weinstein and Stason, 1977; Drummond, 1980; Weinstein, 1981; Drummond, 1981a; Warner and Luce, 1982). The growth and composition of the literature, especially in relation to publication in medical journals, had also been documented by Warner and Hutton (1980) as part of a project commissioned by the Office of Technology Assessment of the US Congress (1980) to assess the methodological status and policy relevance of economic evaluation in the health care field.

In addition, most commentators had found it useful to distinguish between different forms of economic evaluation. *Cost-benefit analysis*, where attempts are made to measure all the benefits in money terms so that these can be made commensurate with costs, was recognised as potentially the broadest form of evaluation. However, failure to measure some of the more intangible benefits of health care programmes (e.g. reduction of pain and suffering) had rendered this approach rather limited in practice and many analysts had preferred to undertake *cost-effectiveness analysis*, where benefits are assessed in the most appropriate physical units such as years of life gained. It was also possible to detect a movement away from a strictly paretian approach to cost-benefit analysis to one which was more concerned with exploring with decision makers the systematic basis for decisions and making values explicit (Drummond, 1981b).

A more recent development has been the growth in the number of cost-effectiveness analyses using a health status or quality of life measure for benefits. This facilitates broader comparisons between health care programmes without the measurement of benefits in money terms (Williams, 1985) and some consider that this development is important enough to give this form of analysis a new label, *cost-utility analysis* (Drummond, Stoddart and Torrance, 1986).

In this chapter the present status of economic evaluation in health care is briefly reviewed and then possible future developments are discussed. This discussion is divided into three areas: developments in commissioning of evaluations, developments in the conduct of evaluations and developments in the use of evaluation results.

PRESENT STATE OF THE ART

Because of the efforts of health service researchers and those who commission studies, the range of application of economic analysis in health care can now be considered to be extensive, although it must be noted that there has been more progress in undertaking the studies than in using the results (Ludbrook and Mooney, 1984). The review undertaken by the US Congress Office of Technology Assessment (1980) identified more than 600 references. It is also clear from one of the most recent reviews (Drummond, Ludbrook, Lowson and Steele, 1986) that most areas of health care activity have been tackled. There have been evaluations of preventive measures as well as curative ones, long-term care as well as high-technology medicine, and drugs and medical devices as well as medical procedures.

There is also general agreement on most of the methodological principles. These are set out in the Department of Clinical

Table 14.1: Ten questions to ask of a published study

1. Was a well defined question posed in answerable form?
   (a) Did the study examine both costs and effects of the service(s) or program(s)?
   (b) Did the study involve a comparison of alternatives?
   (c) Was a viewpoint for the analysis stated or was the study placed in a particular decision-making context?
2. Was a comprehensive description of the competing alternatives given (i.e., can you tell who did what to whom where and how often)?
   (a) Were any important alternatives omitted?
   (b) Was (should) a 'do-nothing' alternative (have been) considered?
3. Was there evidence that the programs' effectiveness had been established?
   Was this done through a randomized, controlled clinical trial? If not, how strong was the evidence of effectiveness?
4. Were all important and relevant costs and consequences for each alternative identified?
   (a) Was the range wide enough for the research question at hand?
   (b) Did it cover all relevant viewpoints (e.g., those of the community or society, patients and third-party payers)?
   (c) Were capital costs as well as operating costs included?
5. Were costs and consequences measured accurately in appropriate physical units (e.g., hours of nursing time, number of physician visits, days lost from work or years of life gained) prior to valuation?
   (a) Were any identified items omitted from measurement? If so, does this mean that they carried no weight in the subsequent analysis?
   (b) Were there any special circumstances (e.g., joint use of resources) that made measurement difficult? Were these circumstances handled appropriately?
6. Were costs and consequences valued credibly?
   (a) Were the sources of all values (e.g., market values, patient or client preferences and views, policymakers' views and health care professionals' judgements) clearly identified?
   (b) Were market values used for changes involving resources gained or used?
   (c) When market values were absent (e.g., clinic space was donated at a reduced rate) were adjustments made to approximate market values?
   (d) Was the valuation of consequences appropriate for the question posed (i.e., was the appropriate type, or types, of analysis — cost-effectiveness, cost-benefit or cost-utility — selected)?
7. Were costs and consequences adjusted for differential timing?
   (a) Were costs and consequences that occurred in the future 'discounted' to their present values?
   (b) Was any justification given for the discount rate used?
8. Was an incremental analysis of costs and consequences of alternatives performed?
   Were the additional (incremental) costs generated by the use of one alternative over another compared with the additional effects, benefits or utilities generated?

Table 14.1 *contd.*

9. Was a sensitivity analysis performed?
   (a) Was justification provided for the ranges of values (for key parameters) used in the sensitivity analysis?
   (b) Were the study results sensitive to changes in the values (within the assumed range)?
10. Did the presentation and discussion of the results of the study include all issues of concern to users?
   (a) Were the conclusions of the analysis based on some overall index or ratio of costs to consequences (e.g., cost-effectiveness ratio)? If so, was the index interpreted intelligently or in a mechanistic fashion?
   (b) Were the results compared with those of other studies that had investigated the same questions?
   (c) Did the study discuss the generalizability of the results to other settings and patient/client groups?
   (d) Did the study allude to, or take account of, other important factors in the choice or decision under consideration (e.g., distribution of costs and consequences or relevant ethical issues)?
   (e) Did the study discuss issues of implementation, such as the feasibility of adopting the 'preferred' program, given existing financial or other constraints, and whether any freed resources could be used for other worthwhile programs?

Source: Department of Clinical Epidemiology and Biostatistics (1984).

Epidemiology and Biostatistics (1984), in the form of a checklist of questions to ask about any published study (see Table 14.1). However, a number of issues still require further debate; these include the relative merits of the different methods of assessing the utility of health states (discussed in this volume by Williams), the pros and cons of including production gains and losses in the cost-benefit model and the consideration of medical care costs in added years of life. This last issue is particularly important in the evaluation of prevention programmes; is it a legitimate cost to a hypertension programme that those whose lives are extended will receive costly treatments for arthritis and cancer in later life, or is the examination of costs and benefits of these treatments a separate issue unrelated to whether or not the hypertension screening programme is mounted?

The recent review by Drummond *et al.* (1986) identified a number of recurring methodological weaknesses in the existing literature. These were:

failure to specify clearly the viewpoint from which the appraisal

189

was carried out (e.g. society as a whole, the public sector, the health care sector);

failure to base the economic study on good medical evidence, such as that generated by controlled clinical trials;

the unthinking use of average costs, particularly in estimating the costs of hospitalisation;

failure to consider patient, family and volunteer costs where these were relevant (e.g in a comparison of community care with institutional-based programmes for the elderly, mentally ill or mentally handicapped;

inadequate allowance for uncertainty in cost and benefit estimation;

inadequate consideration of the link between appraisal results and the decisions, in health service planning and clinical practice, to which they pertain;

failure to consider factors other than economic efficiency (including equity considerations and the managerial procedures required to bring about a change in policy).

If economic evaluation in health care is to progress in the future these deficiencies will have to be resolved. In particular there is a need for a closer understanding between those who undertake studies and those who seek to use the results. Some indications of how these issues might be resolved in the future are given in the next section.

FUTURE DIRECTIONS

Commissioning evaluations

Up until the present time the majority of economic evaluations in the health care field have been undertaken because of the interests of independent researchers. Whilst this is not necessarily a bad thing, very little is known about how individuals formulate their research priorities. No doubt opportunism plays a major role, as well as the individual researcher's perception of the likelihood of a study being published if satisfactorily completed. A major consequence of this situation is that while the methodological quality of studies has greatly improved over the years, there is often no clear link between evaluation results and decisions that have to be taken in health care planning or clinical spheres.

In the future it is likely that more studies will be directly commissioned by interested parties to assist decision making. This will improve both the relevance of the studies that are carried out and the commitment, on the part of decision makers, to use the results. There are already signs that this is beginning to happen. For example, in the United Kingdom the government postponed major decisions on the funding of new heart transplant units until an economic evaluation of the treatments performed by the first two units had been carried out (Buxton *et al.*, 1985).

Also in the United Kingdom, the requirement that health service developments should be formally appraised when one of the options is a capital scheme costing more than £5 million has led to the commissioning of studies by local authorities (Akehurst and Buxton, 1985). Whether such commissioning will spread beyond instances where there is a formal requirement is still open to question. It is to be hoped that local health authorities will consider undertaking or commissioning economic evaluations to inform decisions about large clinical developments, for example.

In other countries, such as the Netherlands, where health services are financed through social insurance schemes, there are also signs that economic evaluation will be more often undertaken in relation to specific decisions, such a whether certain clinical procedures will be allowable for reimbursement (Sturmans and Rutten, 1986). A number of countries are setting up, or considering the establishment of, agencies to assess new health technologies. One aspect of this assessment will be economic evaluation (Drummond, 1986).

The increased interest in economic evaluation by the agencies that fund or plan health care will in turn lead to increased interest by the drugs and medical equipment industries. In the future it will be necessary not only to demonstrate that new products are more effective than those already on the market, but that the additional benefits outweigh any additional cost. Therefore one can expect that industry will undertake or commission evaluations in support of licensing of new products and of pricing decisions. Similarly there are already signs that clinicians wishing to develop new procedures or clinical services are turning to economic evaluation as a way of justifying their claims. This is partly the explanation for the rapid increase in the publication of cost-benefit studies in medical journals.

Whilst in general terms these developments, should they take

191

place, are to be welcomed, three points are worth noting. First, given the slightly differing perspectives of the various parties, it will be increasingly important for economic analysts to be clear on the viewpoint for their study, e.g. does one examine costs and benefits from the point of view of the funding agency, the health care institution or society at large? Indeed there will be an increasingly strong case for examining, in a given study, a range of viewpoints including the societal viewpoint, so that appropriate incentive structures can be devised to facilitate adoption of the socially preferred option. At the present time many economic evaluations merely identify the *potential* for increased efficiency and have nothing to say about the ways of achieving it. This is particularly true of studies examining shifts in the balance of care from institutions to the community, where a number of care agencies (including the family) may experience changes in costs and benefits and require compensation in order to lend their support to the shift in the balance of care.

This leads on to the second point, that whereas the funds for evaluation of high technology, or new drugs and devices, are likely to be readily available, it is important that other areas such as health promotion and care of the chronic sick are not neglected. Indeed the evaluation of changes in lifestyle and other health promotion measures is relatively undeveloped and a number of methodological challenges still remain (Russell, 1986). The same is true for chronic and long term care, where clinical objectives are more concerned with preventing deterioration in the quality of life, rather than extending life. This is one reason why developments in assessing the quality of care (Williams, Chapter 15, below) and the quality of life of informal carers (Mohide *et al.*, 1985) are so important.

Thirdly, it will be important, given the vested interest of various parties, to maintain high methodological standards. Those commissioning research, be they industry or government agencies, have a particular responsibility here. Indeed, given the likely expansion in the number of proposals for undertaking economic evaluations in the future, research funding agencies will need to be clearer on their research priorities and on the appropriate circumstances for undertaking an economic evaluation. The notion of using economic indicators to help develop medical research priorities was discussed some years ago by Black and Pole (1975) but, as far as one can tell, has not been a subject of debate since. The issue of when to undertake an economic evaluation alongside clinical trials was discussed by Drummond and Stoddart (1984), but there are few signs that the bodies funding medical research have insisted that an economic component be added to a clinical research proposal. This may change in the future. Once there is more experience of agencies directly commissioning or encouraging economic evaluations, rather than leaving this to the whims of independent researchers, it may be possible to delineate more precisely the situations where the benefits from undertaking a formal evaluation justify the costs. This issue was discussed briefly by Williams (1974), but as yet there has been no detailed exploration of the cost-benefit analysis of undertaking cost-benefit analysis in the health care field.

Conducting evaluations

In the assessment of the present state of the art given above certain recurring methodological weaknesses were identified. It is likely that in the future many, if not most, of these deficiencies will be resolved.

First, if more economic evaluations are carried out alongside clinical trials or other forms of prospective medical evaluation it is likely that the quality of the underlying medical evidence, upon which studies are based, will improve. Indeed, in the future it will be increasingly rare to see economic studies published by economists alone or, it is to be hoped, clinicians alone! As in other fields the growth of multi-disciplinary working will lead to an improvement in the quality and relevance of the evaluations carried out.

Second, there will be significant improvements in the methods for assessing the utility of health states. This will lead to the increasing ascendancy of cost-utility analysis as the preferred form of evaluation. In particular, it is likely that there will be more thorough testing of data collection instruments, development of visual aids or props to assist respondents in making assessments of the utility of health states, and the exploration of differences in the values of various groups in the community (e.g. doctors, patients, policy makers and the general public). There will also be more discussion of the appropriateness of particular groups' values for particular decisions (Drummond, 1987). It remains to be seen whether 'standard' sets of utility values can be developed for given populations. (Many of these issues are discussed further by Williams in Chapter 15, below.)

Third, there will be developments in the ways uncertainty is handled in economic evaluations, since this is one of the major

193

criticisms of formal analytical approaches (Fischhoff, Lichenstein, Slovic, Derby and Keeney, 1981). The state of the art has improved in recent years and it is now normal for published evaluations to include a sensitivity analysis, where the variation in study results resulting from changes in the values assumed for some of the key parameters is explored. However, most analysts do not give an adequate justification for the range of values assumed, nor the estimates used in the 'base case' or 'most likely' analysis. Also, in presenting a series of estimates (e.g. 'low', 'high' and 'best guess') analysts rarely discuss the *probability* of particular combinations of circumstances occurring. This becomes a particular problem when the sensitivity of results to changes in a large number of parameters is explored. For example, one may produce a very large negative result for a new health care programme if the 'worst case' estimate is used for all of the parameters. Alternatively, it could be argued that if the programme still looks worthwhile under the 'worst case' scenario then the result was so self evident it was not necessary to have undertaken the study!

There have already been some developments in this field. Weinstein (1986) reports attempts to generate the probability distribution for variables through simulation methods. Also, in some studies the probability distribution of some variables, such as length of hospital inpatient stay or patients' travel costs, are measured and statistical tests of significance performed (see, for example, Logan *et al.*, 1981). Finally, some analysts have explored the possibility of using principles of experimental design to assist in developing the strategy for sensitivity analysis in a given study (Goldsmith *et al.*, 1986). Such developments can be expected to continue in the future.

However, a bigger challenge relates to the fact that health service planning takes place under conditions where changes in circumstances may be so uncertain, or so profound, that it is difficult to model them as described above. For example, what would happen to the costs and benefits of (say) options for the location of imaging equipment if there were a significant technological breakthrough or if changes in the funding arrangements for health care meant that physicians could have scanners in their private offices? It has often been argued that analysts have paid little attention to the *robustness* of their results to such changes (Rosenhead, 1980) and there are few good examples of such analysis. Some go as far as to say that formal analyses, like economic evaluation, are of little use in a highly uncertain world. There will always be those who prefer to swim around in a sea of uncertainty. Nevertheless, some progress ought to be made in the future by exploring, with decision makers and the public at large, the appropriateness of different decision making criteria. For example, if the expected value approach, which is implicit in 'standard' economic evaluation, the right one or would it be more appropriate to adopt an approach based on minimising the changes of a major loss? That is, the option which performs reasonably well under all assumptions about the future may not be the one that has the highest net present value under ideal circumstances. In the future there may be more empirical testing in this area, both for health service planning decisions and for individual clinical decisions.

Using evaluation results

It was noted earlier that despite the increase in the quantity and quality of economic evaluations, there is still little evidence of their use in health service planning or clinical decision making. Although this apparent lack of impact should be of concern to economic evaluators, it may be unrealistic to link a given decision with one particular piece of evidence. Decisions in the health care field rightly depend on a complex interplay of social, economic and political factors. The responsibility of economic analysts is therefore to deliver the best quality evidence within the constraints of the resources (including time) available. Indeed a major criticism of economic evaluations is that there are not enough 'quick and dirty' studies producing timely, if not perfect, results. One exception to this was the analysis of the economics of vaccination to prevent a swine influenza epidemic (Schoenbaum, McNeil and Kavet, 1976). In addition, as mentioned earlier it is still possible to find methodologically deficient studies and decision makers have probably done the community a service by trusting their intuitions instead of taking notice of evaluation results. However, there are probably a greater number of instances, typified by the case of the sixth stool guaiac (Neuhauser and Lewicki, 1975), where failure to pay adequate attention to costs and benefits has resulted in an inefficient use of health service resources, with the consequent loss of benefits to the community.

The developments in the commissioning and conduct of economic evaluation outlined above will greatly improve the level of understanding by analysts of decision makers' problems and vice versa. In addition, one may expect more synthesis of evidence from a number of studies in a given area in the future. This will be coupled with a greater understanding by decision makers of the prospects and limitations of economic evaluation, and the methodological quality of individual studies. The evaluation of health care programmes, particularly emerging health technologies, will increasingly be viewed as a dynamic process, where study results are continually updated as new evidence becomes available. This may require more modelling to be undertaken in the field of economic evaluation so a greater number of 'what if?' questions can be asked. There may even be more acceptance of a standardised framework for economic evaluation in health care, as proposed by Russell (1986), so that different analyses of the same health care programmes can be compared, or comparisons made across a range of programmes.

There will also be greater use of the cost-benefit approach as a *way of thinking* about choices in health care and not merely as a basis for undertaking formal studies. This will be greatly facilitated by educational initiatives in the health economics field, especially those for health professionals (WHO, 1986). (Further initiatives are discussed by Buxton, Chapter 12, above.)

In addition, the efficacy of the cost-benefit approach for informing choices in health care will continue to be debated. For example, what is the predictive value of economic evaluations; do costs and benefits turn out as expected in practice? In one well-quoted example from the health and safety field the costs of complying with a new occupational health standard for vinyl chloride monomen turned out to be negative, as compliance with the standard led to the discovery of a more efficient production process involving the recycling of material (Drummond and Shannon, 1986). If decision makers undertake more synthesis of study results through time the reliability of economic evaluations will be better assessed. Also, the moral justification for the use of the cost-benefit approach will continue to be examined (Culyer, 1977; Drummond, 1981b). Is this the most appropriate basis on which to make choices in health care? Can equity considerations be successfully taken into account alongside efficiency data from economic evaluations? To what extent would the community be willing to sacrifice efficiency for the higher *process utility* of particular decision making procedures, especially in the clinical sphere? (For example, would members of the community accept the waste of resources that may be associated with unconstrained clinical activity because as patients they would expect the clinician to be their advocate, rather than to work to guidelines laid down by economic evaluation?) In the planning sphere, would the community wish health care resources to be allocated so as to maximise the number of quality-adjusted life-years gained overall? If not, on what basis would they wish resources to be allocated? These and other issues will be the subject of ethical discussion and, it is to be hoped, empirical study, in the future.

CONCLUSIONS

The discussion above has outlined the development of cost-benefit analysis to its present status and has contained a number of predictions for the future. One further issue merits consideration; could one foresee a future *without* cost-benefit analysis?

It is hard to foresee a world within the next 25 years where resource constraints have less prominence. Therefore the only choice is in how which costs, risks and benefits of health care alternatives are compared, not *whether* they are compared. It may be that with increased multi-disciplinary working the concepts implicit in economic evaluation become assimilated with those from other approaches to evaluation and are not viewed as the sole preserve of economists. Cost-benefit analysis may be called by a different name. Howeer, it would be a brave man who would predict major departures from the fundamental logic implicit in the cost-benefit approach.

REFERENCES

Akehurst, R.L. and Buxton, M.J. (1985) 'Option appraisal in the NHS: a guide to better decision making'. *Nuffield/York Portfolios No. 8*, Nuffield Provincial Hospitals Trust, London.

Black, D. and Pole, J.D. (1975) 'Priorities for biomedical research: indices of burden'. *British Journal of Social and Preventive Medicine, 29*, 222–7.

Buxton, M.J., Acheson, R., Caine, N., Gibson, S. and O'Brien, B. (1985) 'Costs and benefits of the heart transplant programmes at Harefield and Papworth hospitals'. *DHSS Research Report No. 12*, HMSO, London.

Culyer, A.J. (1977) 'The quality of life and the limits of cost-benefit analysis'. In L. Wings and A. Evans (eds) *Public economics and the quality of life*. Johns Hopkins University Press, Baltimore.

Department of Clinical Epidemiology and Biostatistics (1984) 'How to read clinical journals VII: to understand an economic evaluation (Part B)'. *Canadian Medical Association Journal, 130*, 1542–9.

Drummond, M.F. (1980) *Principles of economic appraisal in health care.* Oxford University Press, Oxford.

—— (1981a) *Studies in economic appraisal in health care.* Oxford University Press, Oxford.

—— (1981a) 'Welfare economics and cost benefit analysis in health care'. *Scottish Journal of Political Economy, 28*, 2, 125–45.

—— (1986) *Economic appraisal of health technology in the European community.* Oxford University Press, Oxford.

—— (1987) 'Resource allocation decisions in health care: a role for quality of life assessments?' *Journal of Chronic Diseases* (forthcoming).

—— Ludbrook, A., Lowson, K.V. and Steele, A. (1986) *Studies in economic appraisal in health care.* Vol. 2, Oxford University Press, Oxford.

—— and Shannon, H.S. (1986) 'Economic aspects of risk assessment in chemical safety. *Science of the Total Environment* (forthcoming).

—— and Stoddart, G.L. (1984) 'Economic analysis and clinical trials'. *Controlled Clinical Trials, 5*, 115–28.

—— Stoddart, G.L. and Torrance, G.W. (1986) *Methods for the economic evaluation of health care programmes.* Oxford University Press, Oxford.

Fischoff, B., Lichenstein, S., Slovic, P., Derby, S.L. and Keeney, R.L. (1981) *Acceptable risk.* Cambridge University Press, Cambridge.

Goldsmith, C.H., Gafni, A., Drummond, M.F., Torrance, G.W. and Stoddart, G.L. (1986) 'Sensitivity analysis and experimental design: the case of economic evaluations of health care programmes'. Paper presented at the Third Canadian Congress on Health Economics, Winnipeg.

Klarman, H.E. (1965) *The economics of health.* Columbia University Press, New York.

Logan, A.G., Milne, B.J., Archber, C., Campbell, W.P. and Haynes, R.B. (1981) 'Cost-effectiveness of a worksite hypertension treatment program'. *Hypertension, 3*, 2, 211–18.

Ludbrook, A. and Mooney, G.H. (1984) *Economic appraisal in the NHS: problems and challenges.* Northern Health Economics, Aberdeen.

Mishan, E.J. (1971) 'Evaluation of life and limb: a theoretical approach'. *Journal of Political Economy, 79*, 4, 687–705.

Mohide, E.A., Pringle, D.M., Streiner, D., Gilbert, R. and Roe, D.J. (1985) *An evaluation of a family care giver support program in the home management of demented elderly.* School of Nursing, McMaster University, Hamilton, Ontario.

Neuhauser, D. and Lewicki, A.M. (1975) 'What do we gain from the sixth stool guaiac'. *New England Journal of Medicine, 293*, 226–8.

Office of Technology Assessment of the US Congress (1980) *The implications of cost-effectiveness analysis of medical technology, Background paper 1. Methodological issues and literature review.* Government Printing Office, Washington D.C.

Rosenhead, J. (1980) 'An education in robustness'. *Journal of the Operational Research Society, 292*, 2, 105–11.

Russell, L. (1986) *Is prevention better than cure?* The Brookings Institution, Washington D.C.

Schoenbaum, S.C., McNeil, B.J. and Kavet, J. (1976) 'The swine-influenza decision'. *New England Journal of Medicine, 295,* 4, 759–65.

Sturmans, F. and Rutten, F.F.H. (1986) 'Economic appraisal of health technology in The Netherlands'. In M.F. Drummond (ed.), *Economic appraisal of health technology in the European community.* Oxford University Press, Oxford.

Warner, K.E. and Hutton, R.C. (1980) 'Cost-benefit and cost-effectiveness analysis in health care: growth and composition of the literature'. *Medical Care, 18,* 11, 1069–84.

Warner, K.E. and Luce, B.R. (1982) *Cost-benefit and cost-effectiveness analysis in health care: principles, practice and potential.* Health Administration Press, Ann Arbor, Michigan.

Weinstein, M.C. and Stason, W.B. (1977) 'Foundations of cost-effectiveness analysis for health and medical practices'. *New England Journal of Medicine, 296,* 716–21.

Weinstein, M.C. (1981) 'Economic assessments of medical practices and technologies'. *Medical Decision Making, 1,* 4, 309–30.

——— (1986) 'Risky choices in medicine'. *The Geneva Papers on Risk and Insurance, 11,* 40, 197–216.

Weisbrod, B.A. (1961) *Economics of public health.* University of Pennsylvania Press, Philadelphia.

Williams, A.H. (1974) 'The cost benefit approach'. *British Medical Bulletin, 30,* 252–6.

Williams, A.H. (1985) 'Economics of coronary artery bypass grafting'. *British Medical Journal, 291,* 326–9.

World Health Organization (Regional Office for Europe) (forthcoming, 1987) *WHO study on the development of health economics training: report.* WHO, Copenhagen.

15

Measuring Quality of Life

Alan Williams

WHY ALL THE FUSS?

Medical science and clinical practice have both now advanced to the stage where no country, not even the richest and healthiest, can afford to exploit all the available opportunities to improve the health of its members. In that situation the citizens of each country have to decide how to choose which improvements in health shall be enjoyed by which of their number (a choice which obviously also implies deciding which potential improvements shall be *denied* which of their number). Such decisions may be made explicitly, as part of national policy making, or they may emerge from a myriad of decentralised choices at the level of clinical practice about who shall (and who shall not) have access to particular kinds of health care.

Two criteria seem to dominate discussions of such choices. The first flows from a strongly individualistic stance, in which it is asserted that only the affected individual can judge whether a procedure is or is not beneficial, and how beneficial it is, so that the competition for access to health care should be determined by each individual's willingness to sacrifice other good things in life. This leads to reliance on markets, and on the willingness-to-pay criterion as a means of valuing health benefits. Because of the catastrophic nature of some ill health, and its uneven incidence across individuals and over time, markets for health care are usually dominated by insurance, which diffuses the 'signals' from individuals about what particular improvements in health each of them values most. But the main weakness of this approach is that people's 'willingness' to pay depends also on their 'ability' to pay, and many people feel that differential purchasing power should not be allowed to determine

200

access to health care (or, at any rate, not wholly).

Thus the second major criterion emerges, that of 'need'. This is a rather elusive concept, but generally seems to mean that health care should go to those who will benefit most from it, the judgement about 'benefit most' being made *not* by the individual but by some third party. Thus instead of the valuation of benefits coming from each individual's willingness to pay, it comes from some collective or expert judgement, which is then applied to everybody in a particular state of 'need', irrespective of their particular willingness (and ability) to pay.

In the market (or individualistic) case, individuals require *descriptive* information about how their health will be affected by treatment and will then supply the valuations themselves. For this information they rely mainly on their doctors. The doctor's role is thus to give patients all the information the patient needs in order to make a decision, and the doctor should then implement that decision once the patient has made it. Anyone with the slightest familiarity with the actual practice of medicine will know that it is seldom like that in reality. More often, the roles are precisely the reverse of those indicated above, so that it becomes the patient's role to give the doctor all the information the doctor needs in order that the doctor can make a decision, and the patient should then implement that decision once the doctor has made it. On the whole, doctors do not seem to be very good at conveying to patients precisely what the benefits (and risks) of treatment are, even in a purely descriptive manner, but instead tend to weigh up the advantages and disadvantages in their own heads, and then offer 'advice', of a distinctly prescriptive kind, often on a take it or leave it basis, which the patient (deferring to the authority of the expert) usually accepts. So even in the 'individualistic' case the (implicit) valuations of 'experts' about how beneficial or otherwise a treatment will be seem in practice to play a significant role.

In the need-based (or collective) case, things are no better, because the doctor (as expert) still plays the same role at the point of contact with patients, but may also play the rationing role which is played by ability to pay (or insurance cover) in the market case. By the rationing (or gatekeeper) role I mean controlling access to those treatments which can only be attained by doctor's prescription or by referral from one doctor to another. In a need-based system, the doctor may well be given the explicit task of determining priorities (in the guise of determining 'appropriate' treatment) on behalf of the community generally, including even implementing some notion of fairness when it comes to access to treatment (e.g. not letting people 'jump the queue').

Thus in *all* health care systems there is a need for a great deal more information to be generated and distributed about the prospective benefits of health care, for any or all of the following purposes:

a. to enable individuals to form their own judgements of the relative merits of different courses of action as they affect their own health and welfare;

b. to enable doctors to advise patients on these matters;

c. to enable societies to form a clever view of what their priorities are in deploying whatever resources are available for health care;

d. to enable the actions and decisions of doctors, managers, and policy makers to be better monitored, so that they can more effectively be held accountable to their respective 'clients' (patients, local communities, policy makers, tax payers).

For these reasons I see a very strong prospect that there will be increasingly insistent demands made for better and more widespread quality of life measurement in the next decade.

WHY QUALITY OF LIFE?

When for most people life was nasty, brutish and short (as it still is for some unfortunate people) survival dominated all other objectives. It is still important, but as the average life-span increases, and concern about chronic disabling and distressing conditions looms larger in health care policy, more weight comes to be given to people's *quality* of life. Technical advances in the intensive care of the terminally ill merely dramatise the problem of 'choosing' between quantity and quality of life (and the high cost of such care adds another dimension). Considerations such as these have generated a lively, and as yet unresolved, debate on a variety of ethical, legal, clinical and economic issues about the value of life and when (and by whom) it may be 'sacrificed' (i.e. allowed to terminate) when its quality is so poor as to be unbearable (to the patient and/or his/her nearest and dearest).

It is not my purpose here to embark upon a discussion of those broader issues, except insofar as they are inescapably thrown up by

202

my particular topic, which is the description, measurement and valuation of quality of life in the context of health care provisions. Although I there distinguished 'description', 'measurement' and 'valuation' I do not want to pretend that these distinctions are easy to keep separate in practice, but they are useful distinctions with which to begin.

It is possible to *describe* health (or ill health) in a variety of ways, but since my focus is upon communications between 'experts' and 'patients', and/or between policy makers and citizens, I am seeking descriptions which make sense to ordinary people, and which they can rank in order of importance to them personally, or to people in general. This means starting from ordinary people's own ideas about how they recognise ill health, and what aspects of ill health they are most anxious to avoid. This 'layperson's' approach rules out much biomedical or psychiatric description of ill health, which typically runs either in terms of 'abnormalities' in some parameter or other (e.g. of temperature or blood pressure or haemoglobin count or organ or limb function), or in terms of clinical entities or syndromes (i.e. labelling specific configurations of abnormality which indicate the presence of some known pathological condition — which may or may not be treatable). The 'quality of life' approach to health or ill health is to be sharply distinguished from that clinical approach, because the former concentrates on what patients perceive, and the latter on what doctors need to know to diagnose and treat a patient 'correctly'. Some people think that calling this a 'quality of life' approach claims too much for it, in the sense that there will be some aspects of quality of life (e.g. aesthetic appreciation of architecture, art, music, nature, etc.) which it neglects because they are less salient in the context of health care. This is a fair point, but it is nevertheless a useful way of expressing rather graphically the differences between caring exclusively about 'mere' survival, and caring also about the enjoyment of *good* health.

The aspects of quality of life which seem most important in the context of health are physical mobility, pain and distress, capacity for self-care, and the ability to pursue normal social roles (work, family, leisure). This mixture of feelings and functional capacity is the basic stuff of which most quality of life measurement in the health care field is made. The differences between different measures are mainly to do with the level of detail that is regarded as appropriate, whether a single index is sought or not, and how scaling or valuation is handled.

If the quality-of-life measure is to be used only in a very narrow context (e.g. for patients with one specific condition only) then it can obviously concentrate on those aspects of life on which that particular condition impinges most strongly and ignore the others, and in narrowing the focus may also be able to increase the fineness of the measurements. But if the quality-of-life measurement is to be used to establish an order of priorities across very disparate treatments and conditions, then it needs to be broadly focused, and, for practical reasons of information collection and analysis, will have to suppress detail. This will especially be the case if a single index is sought, requiring explicit relative valuation of all the described states of health, because the number of pair-wise comparisons that might need to be made to establish such an index of value for an individual rapidly reaches unmanageable proportions as categories proliferate (four different levels of 'intensity' for each of four different 'dimensions' of health would generate 256 different combinations, which in turn would generate over 30,000 different pair-wise comparisons of states of health!)

The issue of scaling or valuation is the aspect of quality of life measurement which is most fraught with difficulty. Often the descriptive categories themselves already imply some rank ordering ('mild', 'moderate', 'severe'), or it may already have been established that problems cumulate in a particular sequence, so that if an individual cannot do X, it is most unlikely that he or she could do Y or Z either, so the 'factual' statement that an individual cannot do X already carries the implication that that person is worse off than someone who only cannot do Z. Sometimes people simply add up the number of items on a list to which the respondent gives an adverse response, and that is then used either as a means of rank ordering quality of life, or even as a cardinal measure thereof. Clearly that would only be a valid inference if each adverse circumstance were of equal (negative) value, and if they do not interact with each other (e.g. in a multiplicative way).

It is therefore rather important to be as explicit as possible about the valuation processes built into quality of life measures (as indeed with other conventional measures of benefit, such as five-year survival, return to work, complication or recurrence rates, and so on, which tend to be even more obscure in their valuation implications!).

VALUATION OPTIONS?

There are many different ways of eliciting valuations, each of which has particular strengths and weaknesses (theoretical or practical). The most complex is probably the 'standard gamble', where a respondent is asked to compare two lotteries, one of which offers stated odds of winning a stated prize, the other offering variable odds between two prizes. The respondent is asked to say what the 'variable' odds would have to be for the second lottery to be of identical value to the first. 'Prizes' may be positive or negative, and, in the present context, the 'prizes' would be better or worse health. Most such work in the health field has been concerned with the risk of death (i.e. with survival) not with risks to quality of life.

A different strategy is to pose the choices in terms of the relative amounts of time to be spent in two specified health states, e.g. how many weeks in state A is equivalent to X weeks in state B. If the respondent thinks state A is better than state B, then the 'equivalent' number of weeks on state A will be less than X.

Yet another strategy is to rate directly in numerical terms, the value of a specified health state relative to some specified 'market' state, which has been given a conventional 'value' (e.g. 1). In this approach *two* 'anchor points' might even be used, e.g. that being healthy = 1 and being dead = 0, and all other states are then rated according to this 'scale'. Some states may be negatively rated (i.e. be regarded as worse than death).

There are many interesting variants within each of these broad strategies and we need more systematic comparative work between them. Ignoring the particular technique issues which each throws up, they all raise interesting broader issues to which at present we have only very tentative answers. Amongst these are:

a. Can the different dimensions of health be valued independently and the results subsequently integrated (additively, or multiplicatively, or in some other way) or are the patterns of interdependence so complex that one has to adopt a 'holistic' or 'scenario' approach?

b. Are the relative valuations attached to different states, different according to how long (in absolute terms), you might be in them (e.g. supposing you judged that 2 weeks in state A would be better than 2 weeks in state B, but if it were the rest of your life in A versus the rest of your life in B, would you take a different

205

view of their relative values?).

c. Do people systematically value a given improvement in quality of life available *now* more highly than the same improvement some time off in the future (i.e. do they manifest positive time preference?).

d. Is the value of any particular health state affected by the health states which may precede or succeed it?

e. Are differences in the relative valuations of particular health states between different individuals systematically related to their age, sex, education, occupation, religion, health experiences, etc.

This last point is of particular interest because if systematic differences are present it means that when using such data in the decision making contexts outlined earlier, the issue of whose values are to count in each such specific context will have to be faced explicitly.

There does not seem to me to be a general answer to that (political) question. In dealing with a particular patient in a context in which the patient's own willingness and ability to pay is the accepted criterion for choice, then the clinician's proper task is to conduct the whole valuation exercise himself to elicit the relevant material from the patient. It is unlikely (to put it mildly) that this will be feasible, so the short cut method might be to assume that the patient has the values characteristic of his/her age, sex, education, religion, etc. and offer 'advice' on that basis. But in another situation, such as a health authority deciding whether to expand a facility for elderly stroke patients, should it value the potential benefits according to the views of the population 'at risk' of benefit or according to the views of the people who, say, will consequently be denied better ante-natal care? Or since both groups of potential beneficiaries will be using resources provided by the public at large, should it be the views of the whole (taxpaying) population that should count? Since the health authority is the body with legitimate power to determine priorities, perhaps it should be their own views (or their views of their constituents' views) on the valuation of improvements in health which should dominate.

Fortunately, these consequential political issues are not part of my research agenda, but they do reinforce the need to expand the size of the population on which we have good data concerning the value they place on changes in their quality of life due to health care, for without a much larger number of respondents than we have at present it will not be possible to make the fine distinctions required.

PROSPECTS

Looking forward 20 to 25 years I see a very exciting prospect for significant advance in this field. My optimism is based on the fact that many practitioners see the need for greater attention to, and measurement of, the quality of life of patients, and seem willing to put effort into providing basic data, not only for research purposes, but also because it will be immediately useful to them. The socio-political climate is also one in which greater attention to patients' views and values continues to be a strong factor, and in which, as a consequence, the professions feel that their authority is under threat, and many of them would welcome an opportunity to respond positively and constructively to the demands for greater accountability in terms that make sense to them (such as by showing how much good they are in fact doing for patients). Finally, the economic and financial climate will continue to be one in which there will be increasingly insistent demands for greater efficiency in the provision of health care, and if these demands are not to degenerate into counterproductive cost-cutting which pays no regard whatever to the effects of such cuts on the health of patients, then much better data on such benefits and the value attached to them will be needed.

What I foresee happening therefore is a steady growth in collaborative work between (a) the medical, nursing, remedial, rehabilitative and supportive professions in health care, (b) the epidemiologists, social statisticians and survey research workers and (c) the psychologists, economists and sociologists, all of whose inputs are needed for a balanced corpus of work to develop. Over the next decade developments are likely to continue to be piecemeal and opportunistic, as groups of like-minded people get together to tackle specific problems that they confront, and which interest them sufficiently for the conventional *ad hoc* solutions not to be acceptable. A few people (probably not more than 100 in all in Britain, Canada and the USA, where most of this work is currently concentrated) will make this their main work, but a much larger number will be helping peripherally, though in a crucial way, with data-gathering and applications to different sorts of decision making.

But I also foresee this piecemeal approach becoming increasingly recognised as quite unsatisfactory. Periodically the scattered researchers will get together to assess progress, exchange views, and stimulate each other to greater (or different) effort, and some sporadic co-ordination of activities, and low level standardisations of basic data collection, will slowly emerge, but with different 'schools' offering quite distinct patterns of work. This diversity is no bad thing, since none of us can be sure which approach is going to prove 'best', and it may well be that we need different approaches for different purposes. The problem is going to be that no one group is going to make a big enough impact, by the sheer magnitude of the data base they assemble and the variety of analytical work they can do upon it, for the practical impact of their work to be commensurate with the need for it, as outlined earlier.

If things are left to develop in that serendipitous way, two possible reactions may well set in during the late 1990s. One might be to say: well, we have seen all these people beavering away in their own idiosyncratic ways for over a decade now, and things are still very confused, and all that seems to have been achieved is the recognition that measuring quality of life is fraught with difficulties which are never going to be resolved to everybody's satisfaction, so let's go back to the good old hard end-point of survival or life expectancy, and leave all this 'soft' stuff for people to do *ad hoc* where the situation demands it. That way there will also be less aggro in the system, because it won't any longer be necessary to be explicit about what is happening to patients, and, best of all, it will avoid the unpleasant business of reducing these delicate matters to numbers, which many people feel very uncomfortable with anyway. If that reaction sets in and predominates, the research work will doubtless go on amongst the more visionary and dedicated, but it will be seen as an 'academic' pursuit for a few eccentrics, and far removed from the world of action.

The other possible reaction, in ten years time, might be to say that we should stop pussyfooting around in this business, and launch a massive social survey to get some really representative data on a large number of people (100,000?), such as eventually happened with surveys on poverty, housing standards, educational attainment, etc. To do this will require the various research groups and potential users of the data to come together to reach some sort of consensus as to what would be the most valuable way to use such an opportunity to establish a national data base on the valuation of health. It is the sort of undertaking that would probably take 2 or 3 years to plan, 1 or 2 years to carry out, and the succeeding 5 to digest. It might be a suitable way to mark the year 2000!

But I sincerely hope that we will not actually have to wait that long for such an enterprise to be undertaken, because we need the results of such work right now. A major stumbling block seems to be that the issue is so central to, and pervasive in, the evaluation of health care, that only large funding bodies with long time horizons could tackle it on the scale envisaged, and they tend to be too cautious, preferring to put small sums into small-scale exploratory studies, just as the smaller funding bodies do. No one seems willing to play for the big prize.

Yet there can be no doubt that the greatest gap in our knowledge of the effectiveness of health care is in this field. We have very little systematic knowledge, even of a *descriptive* nature, about the actual effects of most health care on quality of life, and still less on how these effects are valued by the people concerned. It is a constant source of wonder to me that this state of affairs seems to be accepted so calmly, and attempts to remedy it considered so ambitious or expensive, when one considers the quite disproportionate amount of time, energy and money poured into medical and technical innovations *which cannot be properly appraised because we have not tackled the quality of life issues*. A cynic might say 'Ah, there you have put your finger on the explanation', quality of life measurement is too threatening to too many existing activities for there to be any chance of diverting resources away from them into that new, and potentially subversive, enterprise. If the cynics are right then the first of my two supposed late-1990 reactions is the more probable. For the sake of struggling humanity in general, I hope that it is not so.

On a more optimistic note, it is clear that people generally care strongly about their health, and are willing to devote a quite sizeable proportion of their resources to improving it. It would take only a small proportion of those resources to achieve quite remarkable improvements in our current knowledge about the extent and value of such health improvements, and which activities are better at generating them. Sooner, rather than later, I hope someone influential will wake up to this fact, and seize the opportunity to make the measurement and valuation of quality of life the aspect of health care evaluation which comes historically to be recognised as the great achievement of the last quarter of the twentieth century. It is not an impossible dream.

REFERENCES

Two recent compendia contain a very good impression of the nature of the work currently going on in this field:

Culyer, A.J. (ed.) (1983) *Health indicators*. Martin Robertson, London.
Teeling-Smith, G. (ed.) (1983) *Measuring the social benefits of medicine*. Office of Health Economics, London.

Part Four

The Pharmaceutical Industry

16

The Structure of the Pharmaceutical Industry

Frank Münnich

The purpose of this chapter is to analyse the structure of the pharmaceutical industry in two respects. The first part gives a general overview about the current state of the industry. To characterise the overall structure of the industry, five different parameters are examined: production and consumption, market shares, original versus generic products, medical indications and innovations. The presentation is based on readily available statistical data. Here the innovative countries are of special interest. The second part of this chapter tries to make some predictions concerning the industry's future prospects. It includes some general socio-economic developments influencing the worldwide perspectives of the pharmaceutical industry but is primarily a review of factors dominating the current political discussions about cost containment. This is because the future performance of the research-based pharmaceutical industry is likely to be basically dependent on forthcoming decisions in this field.

PRODUCTION AND CONSUMPTION OF AND FOREIGN TRADE WITH PHARMACEUTICAL PRODUCTS

The most important structural characteristic of the pharmaceutical industry is the division between research-based and non-research-based companies. From the regional point of view the innovative firms are situated in the European industrialised nations — mainly in the Federal Public of Germany, France, the United Kingdom, Italy, Switzerland and Sweden — in the USA and in Japan. In 1982 these countries produced 65 per cent of the worldwide pharmaceutical output of about US $94,000 million. On the other hand only

Table 16.1: Production, foreign trade and consumption of drugs 1970 and 1982

	Production % US $ bill			Export % US $ bill			Import % US $ bill			Consumption % US $ bill		
	1982	1970	growth rate	1982	1970	growth rate	1982	1970	growth rate	1982	1970	growth rate
FDR	6.90	1.72	301.2	2.1	0.49	328.6	1.2	0.18	566.7	5.50	1.30	323.1
France	6.50	1.30	400.0	1.6	0.23	595.7	0.7	0.14	400.0	4.35	1.07	306.5
UK	4.50	0.75	500.0	1.7	0.34	400.0	0.7	0.08	775.0	2.85	0.53	437.7
Italy	4.40	0.90	388.9	0.7	0.15	366.7	0.7	0.14	400.0	3.15	0.81	288.9
Switzerland	2.50	0.36	594.4	1.6	0.33	384.8	0.4	0.08	400.0	0.55	0.07	685.7
Spain	0.45	0.12	275.0	0.3	0.04	650.0	0.3	0.07	328.6	0.42	0.15	180.0
Rest of Europe	5.00	1.26	296.8	2.2	0.36	511.1	2.4	0.53	352.8	4.53	2.03	123.2
USA	20.50	6.85	199.3	2.4	0.42	471.4	0.9	0.09	900.0	18.50	6.44	187.3
Japan	15.95	2.83	463.6	0.3	0.07	328.6	1.2	0.22	445.5	12.04	2.89	316.6
Rest of developed	2.60	0.58	348.3	0.3	0.05	500.0	0.8	0.15	433.3	2.62	0.59	344.1
Total — developing	11.05	1.0	1005.0	0.6	0.17	252.9	4.5	1.02	341.2	14.0	2.40	483.3
Total — CMEA	14.00			0.2			0.3			13.0		
World	94.0	17.7	431.1	14.1	2.7	422.2	14.1	2.7	422.2	81.5	18.14	349.3

Sources: 1970 figures, Table 7, *Scrip Yearbook* (1986). 1982 figures, Table 1–4, *Pharma Information* (1982), EEC (1985) *The Community's Pharmaceutical Industry*, Table 3.1, partly own calculations in round figures.

US $47,000 million of drugs were consumed in these countries — about 58 per cent of the worldwide consumption of drugs in 1982. Nevertheless the most rapid increases in production and consumption took place in the Third World during the period of observation (i.e. between 1970 and 1982). Disregarding the consumption-push in Switzerland, the Third World countries clearly have the top position with holding for growth rates of between 1000 per cent and 500 per cent respectively.

The industrialised countries — with the exception of Italy, Sweden and Japan — are also those with a net export surplus. The American pharmaceutical industry holds the top position, as might have been expected, with Switzerland ranking second. Japan, in contrast to her otherwise well-known performance in other world markets, is still a net importer of drugs (see Table 16.1). In the period of observation Japanese exports had one of the lowest growth rates (328.6 per cent) internationally whereas imports, absolutely as well as relatively, grew at a medium rate. Sweden holds the opposite position, showing the highest growth rate as an exporter and the lowest rate of imports.[1] In judging these figures it should be kept in mind that direct flows of goods are losing importance due to a shift of production locations towards the countries of consumption as a result of regulations in these countries.

MARKET SHARES AND CONCENTRATION

The following analysis is not about particular pharmaceutical companies but national pharmaceutical industries.[2] In 1982 the USA and Japan were more or less self-sufficient, the domestic industries holding a domestic market share of 80 per cent and 77 per cent respectively. The Japanese pharmaceutical industry's domestic turnover was 98 per cent of its total turnover, whereas domestic turnover of US firms was only about half that percentage. Italy (78.5 per cent) and France (61 per cent) showed an above-average domestic turnover as well. The rest of the western European pharmaceutical industries vary considerably as far as their domestic or international market shares are concerned. On the basis of these figures it is likely the Federal Republic of Germany, Switzerland and the United Kingdom will keep a fair market share in international drug markets in the future, as is suggested by Table 16.2.

Compared to other domestic industries the national pharmaceutical markets show fairly low degrees of concentration for

Table 16.2: Market shares and turnover shares of selected countries, 1982 (%)

	Market shares in			Turnover shares in		
	USA	Japan	Less developed countries	USA	Japan	Less developed countries
FDR	3.9	4.8	11.5	7.5	8.0	21.0
Switzerland	9.2	2.8	11.0	23.0	5.5	25.0
UK	5.1	1.9	7.5	18.5	5.5	25.0

Source: EEC (1985), p. 115.

companies as well as products. The concentration ratio for the top ten companies in selected countries in 1982 varies between 50 per cent (USA) and 32 per cent (Italy) of the relevant domestic market. Shares in domestic total consumption of the top ten bestselling pharmaceutical products vary from 17.9 per cent (United Kingdom) to 8.3 per cent (FDR). Of course these figures provide only limited information on overall national consumption of drugs as drug markets are extremely heterogenous; i.e. 'the drug market' as such doesn't exist, rather, we have to differentiate between a multitude of independent sub-markets for specific indications.

It is reasonable to assume that concentration ratios for these more narrowly defined markets are well above the given figures especially in 'different' areas like cytostatics. An analysis of the sub-market shares for specific therapeutic groups clearly reveals higher degrees of concentration.[3]

STRUCTURE OF PHARMACEUTICAL PRODUCTS

The supply side of drug markets can be described as follows: there are patent-protected goods as well as so-called generics; most pharmaceuticals are sold on prescription ('ethical drugs'), others are sold freely 'over the counter' (OTC products); drugs are dispensed mainly through pharmacies to the ultimate consumer (Scrip Yearbook, 1986, p. 54). The developments of the last few years, political endeavours to contain costs and the present discussions in health economics suggest that generics and OTC-products are of particular interest. The term 'generics' here covers all imitations of formerly innovative products with active ingredients the patents of which have run out irrespective of their being branded ('branded generics') or not.

In 1984 the highest national market shares of generic products are in Brazil (34 per cent) and Japan (17 per cent). Market shares of generics in European countries seem to be rather modest: Italy 10 per cent, UK 7 per cent, FDR 4.5 per cent and France 2 per cent; in the USA generic manufacturers hold a market share of 17.5 per cent. Additional data are available on the development of the generic market-potential in the USA and the FDR: the German pharmacists association ABDA reckons a market share of about 10 per cent at the end of 1986 (Scrip, 23 June 1986, p. 2ff.). Estimates concerning the USA presume a market share of 25–30 per cent in 1990, a very distinct growth within this five-year period.

Such assessments are based primarily on the time limits of patent-protection on present NCEs and on estimates of future national development in health policies. The vote against an increase of generic substitution in the US state of Connecticut shows (Scrip, 23 June 1986, p. 18), that predictions of a further expansion of generics cannot be based merely on market forces or on an evaluation of cost containment policies. Besides medical and pharmacological considerations on bioavailability and bioequivalence the problem of patients' compliance plays an important role, because a medical treatment based on the cheapest drug may cause mistrust among patients if pharmacists offer drugs of different appearance on different occasions.

Self-medication and consumption of OTC products have risen over the last few years. In 1985 the FDR — Europe's largest national pharmaceutical market — was also the largest European OTC market (18 per cent market share), followed by Italy and the UK (16 per cent and 15 per cent respectively) (IMS, 23 June 1986, p. 9). It is predicted that the total European market in OTC pharmaceuticals will increase in volume from US $14,200 million to US $17,500 million in the period 1985–90, a growth rate of 23 per cent (IMS, 17 Feb. 1986, p. 5). An even more dynamic development — though in the extended period 1985–99 — is estimated for US OTC consumption: it will more than double from US $5,400 million from a possible US $11,700 million (IMS, 12 May 1986, p. 15). In Japan, however, the share of expenditure on OTC products of overall consumption decreased (14.5 per cent in 1975, 8.8 per cent in 1980 and 5.2 per cent in 1984) (IMS, 17 Feb. 1986, p. 15) — a development which is likely to continue. The reasons for this are the small number of efficient OTC products, the general opinion that contacting the GP is safer and cheaper than self-medication and increasing OTC prices due to decreasing OTC sales.

STRUCTURE OF MEDICAL INDICATIONS

Although there are extensive data available, it is difficult to make statistically supported statements about the worldwide structure of indications because the classification of indications differs between different studies. The classification of Table 16.3 shows that anti-biotics and cardiovasculars, the leading groups in terms of demand, will keep their top ranks despite their low growth rates. The highest growth rates are forecasted for cancerchemotherapeutics and anti-arthritics: 50 per cent and 125 per cent respectively during the five-year-period evaluated.

Some hints of likely changes in the structure of indications in selected regions are given in Table 16.4. Data show that only in Latin America — disregarding the demand for steroids — does the consumption increase in all indication groups listed during the decade evaluated, while for North America, western Europe and notably Japan positive growth rates are forecast only for the therapeutic groups of psychotherapeutics and cardiovascular drugs, i.e. indications which customarily are called 'diseases of civilization'.

RESEARCH AND DEVELOPMENT

As stated above a distinctive characteristic of the pharmaceutical industry is its separation into three groups according to the companies policy on research and innovation. Research-oriented companies are typically large companies with high sales volumes. The second group, companies specialising in generic imitations and price competition, is diverse and can be defined only by the marketing approach of its members. While in the USA and UK many generic producers are owned by research-oriented companies, this is not the case in the FDR. The third group with the largest number of companies is made up of diverse producers following quite different production and marketing policies (e.g. developing new formulations, taking licences, specialising in OTC products or in market niches like herbal products or homeopathics).

The first two groups differ dramatically in cost of entry into the

Table 16.3: Estimated demand for drugs by therapeutic group, 1980–2000, in billion US $

	1980 Value	%	1985 Value	%	1990 Value	%	1995 Value	%	2000 Value	%
Antibiotics	8.25	11	11.00	10	18.00	12	28.70	14	40.50	15
Cardiovascular	6.00	8	10.00	9	15.00	10	22.50	11	32.40	12
Antiarthritics	3.75	5	6.65	6	10.50	7	16.40	8	24.30	9
Psychotherapeutics	3.00	4	5.55	5	9.00	6	14.35	7	18.90	7
Analgesics	2.25	3	3.32	3	4.50	3	6.15	3	8.10	3
Cough and cold medicine	2.25	3	3.32	3	4.50	3	5.40	2	5.40	2
Duiretics	1.50	2	2.22	2	3.00	2	4.10	2	5.40	2
Steroids	1.50	2	3.32	3	4.50	3	8.20	4	10.80	4
Oestrogens	1.50	2	2.22	2	4.50	3	6.15	3	10.80	4
Cancerchemotherapeutics	1.50	2	3.32	3	7.50	5	16.40	8	27.00	10
All others	43.50	58	59.08	54	69.00	46	77.95	38	86.40	32
Total	75.00	100	110.00	100	150.00	100	205.00	100	270.00	100

Source: Information Research Limited (1980), p. 82.

Table 16.4: Estimated demand for selected therapeutic groups in specific regions (1980 and 1990)

%

	1980				1990			
	North America	Western Europe	Japan	Latin America	North America	Western Europe	Japan	Latin America
Antibiotics	10.0	12.0	22.6	19.0	8.0	10.0	18.5	20.0
Psychotherapeutic	2.2	7.0	5.4	4.5	7.5	9.5	10.0	6.0
Cardiovascular	8.0	13.0	9.8	4.5	10.0	15.0	13.0	8.5
Analgesics	6.0	5.0	2.0	4.5	7.0	6.0	4.0	6.0
Vitamins	6.8	3.5	8.0	7.0	4.5	2.5	6.0	8.5
Steroids	9.9	7.0	2.9	10.0	11.0	8.5	4.0	7.5
Dermatologicals	2.7	5.0	3.8	2.8	2.5	4.0	2.5	2.5
All others	54.7	47.5	45.5	47.7	49.5	44.5	42.0	41.0
Total	100.0	100.0	100.0	100.0	100.0	100.0	100.0	100.0

Source: Information Research Limited (1980), p. 82.

market. This is due to the high cost of research and development and the difficulties of setting up a new line of research, especially in acquiring the necessary human capital. In contrast, setting up to produce generics is extremely simple, especially when the effective ingredient is available on the market as bulkware. This could have far reaching consequences for the stability of the market.

Table 16.5: R&D expenditures for drugs

Country	National R&D expenditure (in million US$)			National R&D expenditure (as % of sales)		
	1975	1982	Growth rate (%)	1975	1982	Growth rate (%)
FDR	294	900	206	6.6	13.0	97
France	184	700	280	6.5	11.0	69
UK	175	600	243	11.3	13.2	17
Italy	113	230	104	5.1	5.3	4
Switzerland	244	344	41	—	—	—
Spain	47	—	—	18.8	—	—
USA	991	1818	83	9.9	—	—
Japan	317	960	203	5.2	—	—

Source: Pharma Info (1982), Table 6; EEC (1985), p. 47; Scrip Yearbook (1986), p. 45; partly own calculations.

At the same time the R&D cost per NCE has risen considerably (see Table 16.5). The available data show that R&D expenditures grew considerably in the period observed, not only in absolute figures but in relation to national sales as well. The large growth of R&D expenditure in relation to turnover — in real terms — can be interpreted as an increased effort for innovation. It is estimated that in order to stay in business annual R&D expenditure in the order of US $40 to 50 million is required, i.e. in terms of sales, about US $250 to 350 million. The scale of operations explains the closed-shop character of the top (research-oriented) of the industrial structure and shows why the ten best-selling European pharmaceutical manufacturers of 1982 (with one exception) were identical with those in 1977 and even in 1972 (EEC, 1985, ch. 5.2).

PROSPECTS FOR THE FUTURE: GENERAL ASPECTS

Future structural changes in the international pharmaceutical industry are dependent on developments in a broad range of

Figure 16.1: World pharmaceutical consumption

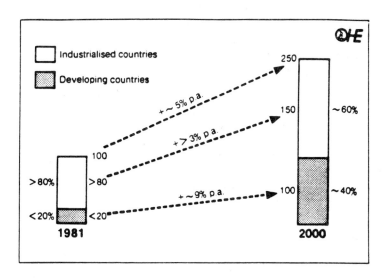

Source: Nowotny, 1983, p. 59.

economic, social and political factors (Nowotny, 1983; Bezold, 1981). On the one hand there are factors likely to generate positive influences, for example the increase of population, longevity, economic progress (especially in developing countries), increasing access to drugs, the invention of better or even breakthrough drugs and, last but not least, the introduction of new technologies. On the other hand there are as many negative factors: price and volume controls, rising cost of research, delays in registration policies linked with a weakening of patent protection and the attack on brand names. It should be noted that these latter factors mainly, if not exclusively, hamper the development prospects of the research-based pharmaceutical industry.

According to the data in Figure 16.1 overall pharmaceutical consumption is expected to grow by 150 per cent by the year 2000. The annual growth rate of about 5 per cent can be split up into annual rates of roughly 3 per cent for industrialised countries and roughly 9 per cent for developing countries.

First estimates on worldwide demand for drugs seem to show further growth: in terms of 1980 US$ the value of worldwide consumption is expected to grow to US $15,000 million in 1990,

221

US $205,000 million in 1995 and US $270,000 million in the year 2000 (Information Research, 1980; Rahner, 1986; Scrip, 4 June, 1986). This implies a growth rate of about 33 per cent for each five-year period. It is to be expected that the relative rate of growth will remain positive but will decline overall.

The overall figures hide large differences between regions and countries. Absolute as well as relative growth figures show that European drug markets increasingly lag behind the fast developing world market, especially in comparison with the USA and Japan. The double digit growth rates in Latin America and Africa — continuously between 10 per cent and 13 per cent — are of particular interest. The growing importance of the densely population developing countries is obvious; their share in worldwide demand will double by the year 2000 from roughly 10 per cent at present.

Disaggregating the regional structure by splitting it into national drugmarkets turns out to be of particular interest. With an estimated growth rate of 175 per cent the Japanese domestic demand for pharmaceutical products will nearly triple, whereas that of Brazil (growth rate 378 per cent) will possibly quadruple; developments in a similar range are estimated for Mexico and South Korea.

PROSPECTS FOR THE FUTURE: STRUCTURAL CHANGES

Seven different developments which will be responsible for most of the structural changes expected to take place within the next two or three decades may be singled out:

1. A partial satiation of markets in developed countries as opposed to increasing absolute and relative importance of the less developed Third World countries especially those in the upper income brackets of the World Bank category 'middle income countries'.

2. The changing age distribution of the population of many high-income countries with increasing proportions of aged and super-aged.

3. The changing distribution of the incidence of different diseases which is partially related to the above-mentioned causes.

4. The increasing importance of cost-containment measures, especially to protect publicly mandated social insurance schemes

against the ever increasing demands of sick people and the income expectations of a growing number of suppliers.

5. The imminent revolution in production technology.

6. The persisting and even accelerating increase in R&D cost which is largely due to the last two causes mentioned and to an ever increasing desire for safety.

7. Changes in attitudes.

These developments are discussed in turn.

1. The increasing importance of Third World countries has several profound implications, stemming from their specific socio-economic characteristics, mainly their low income level. Despite the better economic performance of many of these countries they cannot and, for some time will not, be able to afford costly pharmaceuticals in quantities of the order of present consumption in developed countries. This is due on the one hand simply to a general lack of funds and especially to a lack of hard currencies. On the other hand, different equally urgent needs like investment in productive capital or crude oil as a source of primary energy, compete successfully with health goods for sparse foreign exchange.

Two effects are obvious. The first is a diversion of trade flows. The research-oriented companies in the most developed countries demanding high prices to finance their research efforts will lose market shares to either generic producers in the same countries or to low price producers from less developed 'borderline' or Comecon countries.

The second consequence will be a decrease in the average worldwide prices of pharmaceuticals and therefore a decline in the rate of return on investment in research. Specifically, the orphan drug problem will be aggravated. Research efforts will be concentrated more and more on the diseases of rich people with high rates of incidence and tropical diseases, despite their high incidence, are likely to be neglected.

Increasing local demand will spur the development of national and supranational regulations. But the national regulatory agencies will not be able to enforce their regulations effectively in many cases because of poor bureaucratic organisation as well as lack of funds and specific competence. Therefore the WHO will step in and gain an ever growing importance as a worldwide regulatory institution.

223

Besides its direct importance for and within Third World countries the WHO will influence the climate of legislation in the developed countries of the leading research-based companies. Worldwide consumer groups will add further momentum to this development. The thrust of all these endeavours will be the implementation of an essential drug list, low-cost provision of the drugs needed (perhaps through price negotiations or tender), effective surveillance of adverse drug effects, and the development of a national if not nationalised 'home industry' in the Third World.

The ultimate result may be a completely different overall geographical pattern of production and consumption and possibly the emergence of a homogeneously regulated world market for pharmaceuticals. The market itself will not be homogeneous as further considerations show.

2. While developing countries will show high rates of reproduction for quite some time — their birth rates will slow down only gradually — the highly developed pharmaceutical markets are experiencing a dramatic drop in population growth. The latter developments augur profound changes in age distribution, the aged and even super-aged (above 85) gaining in relative importance. Older people typically need more, more varied and different prescriptions than younger people. The cost of an average prescription for someone aged 70 is approximately five to seven times higher than for someone aged 20. Typically the elderly suffer from several diseases at once which may all be treated with pharmaceuticals, and their diseases differ markedly from those of younger people.

An aging population therefore has a strong impact on the volume and the structure of prescriptions. This in turn influences the direction of research towards cardiovascular diseases, malignant neoplasms and general age-induced degenerations.

It may happen that the world market will be split into a high-income segment with a fair range of novelties geared towards the 'old-age sicknesses' on the one hand and a low-income segment with a very restricted number of well-established 'old' and cheap products from many diverse sources.

3. The predominant diagnoses differ markedly between 'rich and old' countries on the one side and 'poor and young' countries on the other side. Furthermore the climate and other natural differences contribute to this differentiation. Diseases well under control in western Europe, e.g. tuberculosis, are still a major cause of

mortality in developing countries as are tropical parasitic diseases. In addition there are as yet unexplained changes in the rates of incidence of several diseases. All these may influence the future pattern of products in an unpredictable way.

4. Another major cause of structural change will be the cost-containment policies to which all developed countries have committed themselves. The adopted policies and the measures pursued are as diverse as the political climates of these countries. Nevertheless two different types may be distinguished, although they are not to be found in pure form in any country. One approach might be termed 'competitive'. It rests mainly on strengthening generic substitution by physicians or pharmacists. The USA and Germany may be taken as examples.

The other approach favours price negotiations between producers and third party payers or even a direct price-setting scheme. In the case of countries with important research-oriented companies these measures may be supplemented by measures allowing R&D-cost to be passed on in prices. An example of this case is the UK. Evidently while the latter measure protects research within the national border, the former ultimately poses a threat to the research-oriented industry.

As political decisions are especially difficult to predict, the real impact of the pressure for generic substitution is open to speculation. It could well happen that as generic substitution becomes more and more effective, European countries will become more aware of its double-edged effects and the political pressure will fade.

Also, the industry's own reaction must be considered. The big research-based companies endure large losses in sales and profits without fighting back. Most probably they will try to gain complete control over the generic business themselves and a strong tendency towards concentration may result. Thus, the final outcome cannot even be guessed at.

5. The imminent change in production and research technologies will be of great importance. The chemical procedures dominant now will give way to biochemical and gene-technological methods. This will be true for therapeutic devices as well as for diagnostic ones. The final degree to which the latter will substitute for the former and the speed of this development are as yet unclear. It looks as if some expectations of the potential of the new technologies were/are exaggerated. No real breakthroughs in efficacy, safety or cost have been

made by the first new products (like insulin). If the development gains momentum and gets a real take-off it may change the geographical and national pattern of the industry tremendously.

Due to the advances of American and Japanese companies the traditional importance of Swiss, British and German companies may be reduced. Another profound change may be on the horizon. Experience in other industries suggests that new technological stages are quite often put into practice by newcomers first, not by the well-established leaders of the former stages. This need not necessarily change the structure of the industry, but it might lead to a switch of the relative positions of different firms.

6. Stricter regulations, diminishing returns for research in traditional areas, a switch to the extremely expensive gene-technology, and pressure on market prices and large economies of scale, all these factors will increase competition among research-based enterprises and eventually result in the elimination of the less successful ones. Thus we expect a second dichotomy to emerge in the market with extremely large international research-based conglomerates on the one hand and small, highly specialised units catering to local markets only on the other.

7. Finally the possible importance of developments in the attitudes and behaviours of physicians as well as scientists and of patients should be emphasised. They are increasingly critical of the paradigm of scientific medicine, unchallenged up till now, and are seeking alternatives. Although these alternatives are neither neatly defined or specified and the critics are not agreed among themselves, it is fairly obvious that they all doubt the usefulness of the present prescription and consumption patterns of pharmaceuticals.

They may be even more critical of gene-technological products. If they are even moderately successful, they will not only depress the growth rate of the industry but also may induce some important structural changes towards more 'pre-scientific' drugs.

FINAL REMARK

Thus the general picture looks rather dim. It is not so much the endogenously produced trend — that looks quite promising — it is the political setting which endangers the industry's future. Yet there is hope. As trained economists we know that predictions do not foreshadow the future but are intellectual challenges to change the existing course of events.

Having done the job I was asked to do, I must confess that I am myself a critic of the science of predicting, and a nostalgic admirer of evolution and progress, the course of which cannot be predicted by prophets of any kind but is shaped by the interplay of thousands of activities of those who do it. Let's take part in it.

ACKNOWLEDGEMENT

Valuable help in preparing this chapter was given by Dr Michael Wiegand. He and Ludwig Merz also prepared parts of the translation. All remaining errors are mine.

NOTES

1. For a compilation of the data on the structure of and trade in the pharmaceutical industry in the period 1970–82 see Office of Health Economics (1985), pp. 11–15.
2. Cf. EEC (1985).
3. Dispensation through doctors and hospitals is not taken into account in this context.

REFERENCES

Bezold, C. (1981) *The future of pharmaceuticals — the changing environment of new drugs*. Wiley Medical, New York.
EEC (1985) *The community's pharmaceutical industry*. Luxembourg.
IMS Pharmaceutical Newsletter (1986) 'Japan's OTC market continues to stagnate'. 17 Feb.
—— (1986) 'Prospects for European OTC and specialities markets'. 17 Feb.
—— (1986) 'US OTC drug market set to grow to $12 billion by 1994'. 12 May.
—— (1986) 23 June.
Information Research Ltd. (1980) *Opportunities for pharmaceuticals in the developing world over the next 20 years*. London.
Nowotny, O. (1983) 'Europe: the economic challenge'. In N. Wells (ed.), *The second pharmaceutical revolution*. London.
OHE (1985) *Pharmaceuticals in seven nations*. London.
Rahner, E. (1986) 'Ungebrochene Dynamik des Welt-Pharmamarktes — stagnation in Europa wird immer deutlicher'. *Die Pharmazeutische*

Industrie, 48, 6, 567ff.

Scrip no. 1108 (1986) 'Japan, "internationalise or die"'. 4 June, p. 20ff.

—— no. 1113 (1986) 'Connecticut votes against generic legislation'. 23 June, p. 18.

—— no. 1113 (1986) 'FDR no longer generic "promised land"'. 23 June, pp. 2–4.

Scrip Yearbook (1986) PJB Publications, Richmond, UK.

17

Pricing Medicines

Klaus von Grebmer

BASIC ASPECTS

Pharmaceutical therapy has to be regarded as a factor securing health. In the past, the partial dominance of either industrial or social policy has often hindered a sound synoptic health economic approach to optimally priced medicines.

The pricing of medicines seen in the context of health economics, addresses three basic questions (see Feldstein, 1979):

allocation of resources (which resources should be spent on health products and services and how should these services be composed?)
optimal production (how can health be efficiently secured both technically and economically?)
distribution (how should health services be distributed among the population?)

These basic questions can only be answered within a given political framework so they are automatically structured by the political system. Systems favouring private initiative and allocation of health resources including price mechanisms will reach different answers from the more socialised systems which prefer non-price allocation methods. Thus, the economic question of pricing medicines has to be viewed within the framework of political goal-setting and goal-achieving processes.

'Economics does not tell which competing goals should be adopted. But economic analysis can help to determine if a particular measure contributed to stated goals and at what cost.' (Lipsey and Steiner, 1978). The question, therefore, of how a pharmaceutical market should be organised to contribute efficiently to health care cannot be answered in a general way. Nevertheless, a sound analysis is of increasing importance. Recent research has shown that among factors affecting health care (e.g. hospital care, physicians' services, medical therapy) the highest productivity increases have originated and will continue to originate from technological advances in drug therapy (Stahl, 1979). Therefore, a pricing policy providing an innovative climate as well as a form of workable competition within the pharmaceutical market could be an efficient health and industry policy option.

PARTICULARITIES OF THE PHARMACEUTICALS MARKET

The pricing policy of the pharmaceutical industry — with its unique particularities — cannot be compared with that of the classical product market. Thus, an analysis of pricing policy activities of this industry — utilising the usual economic competition-policy instrumentation — is limited. Neither the classical economic theories i.e. 'non-restricted', 'monopolistic' or 'restricted' competition nor the new concept of 'workable' competition fully take into account the complexity of the pharmaceutical market (Clark, 1940; Chamberlin, 1933).

The classical theory of suppliers' behaviour concentrates only on price competition, thus neglecting the aspects of research-, quality- and information-competition, all of which are of the utmost importance to the pharmaceutical market. To date a generally accepted oligopoly-theory has not been developed. A basic competition-policy — existent only as an approach — would ensure that the prevailing oligopolies were taken into account in the therapeutical sub-markets. Prices for products and services depend on given particular markets. However, seen from the economics point of view the various medicines — due to their product-specific indications — subsequently lead to relevant therapeutical sub-markets.

The essential peculiarities of the pharmaceutical market are the result of several factors:

(a) the characteristic three-tier demand system: the physician prescribing the product; the patient taking it; and health insurance picking up the tab. The alleged economic inefficiencies of this specialty market have led to government interventions. On the one hand, consumers in this particular market, both physician and patient, bear only a small part of the costs — if any — thus they do not have any particular interest in the most economical therapy. On the other hand, health insurance merely has to cover the costs. From this it follows that the demand for medicines can have low price-elasticity and thus does not conform with market-price-principles.

(b) The high costs of research and development of the research-based industry to date amounting up to approximately SFr Mio 100–300 for every newly-introduced medicament (Langle *et al.*, 1983). This paramount feature of the pharmaceutical market accounts for intertemporal allocations as well as a specific cost structure.

(c) The internationality of the research-based supplier coupled with the problem of country-specific allocation for R&D expenditures.

(d) Non-transparency of supply due to the multitude of pharmaceutical products.

(e) Oligopolistic structure of supply in therapeutical sub-markets.

(f) Deliberate limited competition through ban of comparative competition, intervention in pricing and price adaptations of new products, legal restrictions of drug substitutions by the pharmacist, restrictions on practising physicians' freedom, controlling hospital-constructions and -infrastructure etc.

Due to the above particularities the government has intervened in the pricing-policy activities of the pharmaceutical industry in most countries.

RESEACH COST ALLOCATION PROBLEMS

The pricing problems for pharmaceutical products would be much reduced if society were satisfied with the drug therapies available. Today's problems arise from the intensity of research and the international division of labour. Research means an intertemporal allocation of costs: people have to pay today for research expenses which may bring better drug therapies tomorrow. As long as society is ready to pay higher prices for new and better drug therapies this intertemporal allocation process can remain privately organised. If

231

this readiness ceases research either has to be organised publicly or it will stop. Another problem, which will only be touched in this chapter, is the international allocation of research costs. Research today takes place only in a few countries. Nevertheless, the results of it are sold worldwide. If the recipient countries do not pay for it in accordance with the therapeutic benefit which they obtain from the supplying countries, research funds will shrink.

These problems, have already been dealt with in other industries:

> What is the proper place of competitive forces in promoting innovation or dealing with it, and how may they take their proper place and render effective service? As to this there is probably no problem area in which monopolistic and competitive features are so inseparably interwoven. These include patents and their expiration, uniqueness and efforts to imitate it, differential advantages and the competitive erosion of them (Clark, 1961).

Introducing the size of a firm as an addition problem. Penrose stresses:

> Here is the basic dilemma: competition is the essence of the struggle among the large firms that induces and almost forces the extensive research and innovation in which they engage and provides the justification for the whole system; at the same time the large firms expect reward for their efforts, but this expectation is held precisely because competition can be restrained (Penrose, 1968).

PRICING AND COST STRUCTURE

To discuss the pricing methods of pharmaceutical companies, wherein lies the key factor to allocation of resources to the industry and their distribution among the participants, one has to recognise the nature of prices. This is especially true for the prices of pharmaceutical products, which have a number of dimensions as shown in Figure 17.1. 'Price competition takes place therefore among manufacturers in their competitive striking on all the dimensions of the product's quality, since changes in quality change the actual price' (Weston, 1979). There is no possibility of cost-oriented pricing for research-intensive pharmaceutical companies. Nevertheless, the knowledge of the specific cost structure of the research-based

Figure 17.1: Dimensions affecting price

Quality =	Efficacy
	Safety
	Clinical evidence
	Experience
	Information communicated to doctors and other professionals
	Reputation of manufacturer based on performance of prior products
Nominal price =	Price to wholesaler
	Discounts to wholesaler
	Discounts and rebates to hospitals or other distribution outlets
Factual price =	Nominal price in relation to quality

companies is the key to understanding their market behaviour when considering their pricing strategies, the competition and their conduct in the market place. The cost structure can also help to explain the competitive process between research-based companies and non-research-based companies.

The activities of research-based pharmaceutical companies cover, besides other industrial functions, the following main fields: production of new knowledge (by research and development); the diffusion of new knowledge (by medical information and marketing); the manufacture of physical goods. The typical cost structure for research-based and non-research-based companies (see e.g. Slatter, 1977) is shown in Figure 17.2. The research-intensive companies can allocate directly to an individual product only a small fraction of their costs. It is important to note that even the 40 per cent production costs are a *consolidated average*: individual drugs may have products costs of 10 per cent or less of their selling price. Empirical

233

Figure 17.2: Cost-structure: innovator-imitator (% of total turnover)

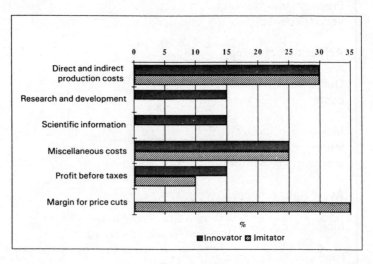

data show that in a research-based company, on average, not more than 30 per cent of the costs can be allocated directly to individual products, the remaining costs and the profit margin have to be covered by contributions (i.e. the difference between the selling price and direct attributable costs) from total sales of the whole product range.

PRICING STRATEGIES

The consequences of this cost structure are that the manufacturer cannot use the *cost-plus approach* (see Rosenberg, 1977, p. 350) for a single product price = direct costs + overhead costs + profit margin. The research-based company's approach to pricing has therefore to be market-oriented. The manufacturer compares the benefits of his products (higher safety, fewer side-effects, higher efficacy, better patient compliance, etc.) with those of the drug therapies already on the market. The greater his additional benefits are, the higher he can price his products above the already marketed drug therapies — but he does not necessarily do so. Normally he has two possible strategies in pricing his new product: skimming pricing or penetrating pricing (see Simon, 1982).

Skimming works best when there is little chance of competitors

Figure 17.3: Skimming pricing

> Preparations to which the consumer does not react very susceptibly to the price (= low price elasticity)
>
> Achieving short-term profits
>
> Quick amortisation of research and development costs
>
> Making profits in the early phases of the products' life cycle (= reducing the risk that new, better preparations contribute to loss of profit)
>
> Avoiding the necessity of price increases
>
> Margin for price reductions
>
> High prices signalise high quality
>
> Limited production possibilities

Figure 17.4: Penetration pricing

> Preparations to which the consumer reacts very susceptibly to the price (= high price elasticity)
>
> Achieving fast quantity growth
>
> Achieving high market share and thus strong market position by the time of competitors' entry
>
> Utilisation of experience curves ('learning curves') and of magnitude advantages in production ('economies of scale')
>
> Low introductory prices reduce risk of a flop
>
> Hindering potential competitors to enter the market

235

entering the market quickly, especially when the product is protected by a patent. This advantage must be balanced against the extra incentive a high skimming price may give to competitors to speed up their entry plans (Rosenberg, 1977, p. 350) (see Figure 17.3). The penetration approach calls for a price low enough to get the product as deeply into the market as possible, establish brand loyalty, and keep two steps ahead of the competition. Penetration may be instituted as a strategy at the time of the product launch or it may follow a skimming period (Rosenberg, 1977, p. 367) (Figure 17.4).

It may also be that the pricing of pharmaceuticals — due to the impossibility of a full cost calculation — follows 'competition-oriented pricing', an approach which has not yet been thoroughly empirically investigated.

One of the easiest methods of pricing is to base your price on what the competition is charging. This does not necessarily mean to charge the same as the competition — many companies will try to keep their prices a set percentage above or below competition. The distinguishing characteristic of competition oriented pricing, however, is that the prime relationship is not between price and cost or demand. Costs may vary, but the company tries to keep its price in line with competitors. The firm assumes, usually quite logically, that the average price level represents a reasonable one (Rosenberg, 1977, p. 361).

If this actually were the main strategy, government interventions on single drug prices could start price wars. This could, in the long run, damage all but the strongest companies in the market.

FINANCING RESEARCH VIA PRICES

Today pharmaceutical R&D expenses are financed by the consolidated contributions of new and old products, products with high and low sales, patented as well as non-patented products. According to this method each product contributes the same percentage to R&D costs — the successful products, however, with higher absolute amounts.

This form of financing is common in the industry and will work as long as research-based companies are not forced by interventions to lower their prices of non-patented products to the price level of non-research-based companies. If this happens, research-based

Figure 17.5: Possible outcome of changes in the market conditions

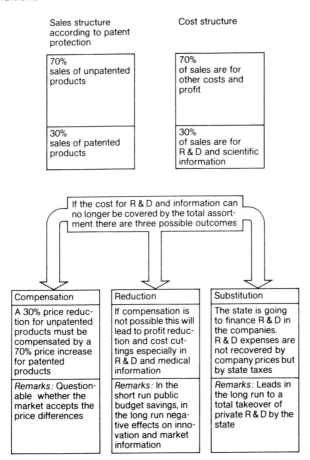

companies would have to recover their total R&D costs from revenue raised from those products still under patent. This would lead to large increases in the prices of patented products, with the long-term result that this additional cost would not be paid by the sickness funds, because other drug therapies were available at much lower prices. Progress in drug therapy does not generally happen in large steps but only in small ones. So, if a product which is still patented is much higher priced than a non-patented product, this may not automatically correspond to differences in the therapeutical benefits as seen by the consumers. This situation would therefore

237

lead to a reduction of R&D funds. If this reduction is not wanted by society, the state would have to take over the financing of R&D. Figure 17.5 shows the possible outcomes.

HETEROGENEOUS COMPETITION

The research-based company has a certain degree of freedom to choose the price of its new product. The actual price strategy will depend on the competitive situation, the expected life-time of the product in question, the estimated time-lag after which competitors may appear on the market, etc. The consumer is protected against exploitation by the fact that, even with new and patented products there are always other drug therapies available as substitutes (actual heterogeneous competition). The market is transparent enough not to accept high price differentials from low innovations (see Reekie, 1977; 1978). If one measures this heterogeneous competition by changes in the rankings of research-based companies, this gives the results shown in Figure 17.6 for the ten leading companies worldwide.

Figure 17.6: Ranking order of the leading international pharmaceutical companies

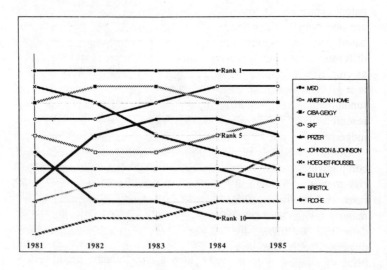

HOMOGENEOUS COMPETITION

At the end of the patent protection the imitators (i.e. non-research based companies) enter the market place, if — and only if — the product in question is still interesting from a profit point of view. The non-research-based companies initiate homogeneous competition and thus reduce the 'pioneering' profits of the innovating companies. The innovator is forced to discover new and better therapies if he does not want to lose his place in the competitive process.

The research-based company can defend its market position after patent expiration by price reducing. Such a strategy involves the danger that the research-based company ties up more and more human and capital resources within this 'imitative market' and thus weakens its competitive capacity in the 'innovative market' where heterogeneous competition still continues. Nevertheless, there are empirical examples where research-intensive companies have met the lower prices of the imitators. Upjohn's price for Neomycin went down from $0.60 per tablet in 1952 to less than $0.20 in 1963 (Bureau of Consumer Protection, 1979). The number of sellers in that market increased from 1 (Upjohn) to 18.

More common in the industry is the attitude of research-based companies letting themselves be 'priced out' of the market after patent expiration. In that phase of the market high price differentials are observed between the products of research- and non-research-based companies. Even without any state intervention, these price differences have led to constantly decreasing sales of the innovator, as empirical examples prove. It is not clear whether the innovator is at all in a position to meet the imitator's price. There are several fundamental structural differences between research-based and non-research-based companies which do not allow an easy economic judgement. Figure 17.7 shows these main structural differences.

One of the basic structural differences is that the research-based company has to recover its services and 'sunk costs', including a fair risk-premium through its physical products, whereas the non-research-based competition really only has to recover the costs of manufacturing and distribution. When considering the empirical data from Germany, for example, the imitator (if he does not dispense medical information) can easily undercut the innovator's price by more than 35 per cent and make an even higher profit on his (lower) capital investment than the innovator. The cost structure of non-research-based (but medical information supplying)

Figure 17.7: The two pharmaceutical markets

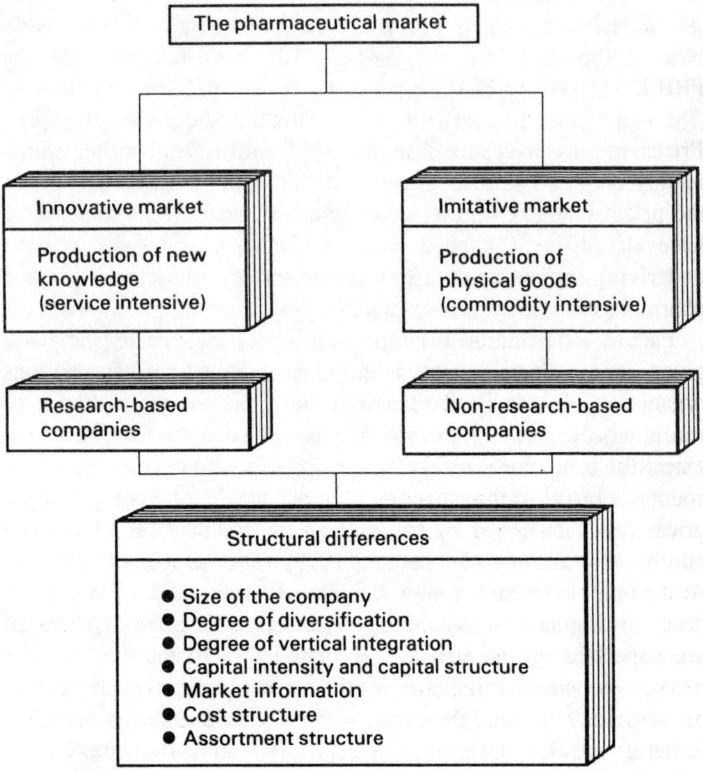

companies makes this apparent (see Figure 17.2 bottom circle).

A sound combination of homogeneous and heterogeneous competition works to the benefit of society. The consumer gets new therapies, he has a choice between different products and the market mechanism is not distorted by government interventions. If the conditioning factors of the market or direct governmental interventions give undue advantage to the non-research-based firm (via bias towards social aspects of low drug prices), this distortion may lead, in the long run, to the detriment both of further progress in drug therapy and of productivity increases in health care. Considered from an industrial policy and pricing point of view, there is strong evidence that in many countries the interventions in a hitherto more or less balanced competitive process have gone or are going in the wrong direction. It may well be that the existing 'second best' solution is superior to any changes which might emerge from trying to enforce other competitive parameters.

PRICE TO THE PUBLIC

Prices of pharmaceuticals to the public are often controversial, mainly because of obvious national and international differences in the prices charged for pharmaceuticals. A wide variety of studies have already been carried out in order to examine the reasons underlying international differences of prices to the public in the pharmaceutical sector.

Factors determining prices to public for pharmaceuticals in a given country consist chiefly of the form in which its market is organised (i.e. whether the market is based on private enterprise or run along the lines of a centrally planned economy), and to what extent the state intervenes in the market as well as the nature of the country's social insurance system. Under ideal circumstances, drug prices are determined by the process of competition and by the purely economic interplay between the forces of supply and demand. At the other extreme is the situation in which the prices charged for drugs, including those which the manufacturer is entitled to charge, are stipulated by the state. At the risk of oversimplification, the markets on which drug manufacturers are currently operating may be said to fall into three categories: 'free market economies' (criteria: price competition, supply and demand mechanisms), 'mixed market economies' (criteria: indirect market control) and 'regulated markets' (criteria: state control, cost curbing). These three categories are, of course, merely models. It should be noted that in reality the distinctions between these categories tend to be somewhat fluid. Although prices to the public for pharmaceuticals are subject to a wide variety of different political, administrative and economic market conditions, nearly all countries have one common denominator relevant for differences in price to the public: the system for the distribution of drugs on the various national markets is laid down by the national authorities, whose stipulations are legally binding. What influence these margins exert on the level of drug prices in various countries is illustrated in Figure 17.8.

241

Figure 17.8: Price structure of a prescription drug supplied by the manufacturer at a price of 10 DM

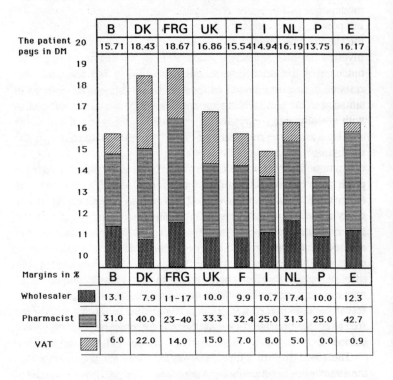

	B	DK	FRG	UK	F	I	NL	P	E
The patient pays in DM	15.71	18.43	18.67	16.86	15.54	14.94	16.19	13.75	16.17

Margins in %	B	DK	FRG	UK	F	I	NL	P	E
Wholesaler	13.1	7.9	11–17	10.0	9.9	10.7	17.4	10.0	12.3
Pharmacist	31.0	40.0	23–40	33.3	32.4	25.0	31.3	25.0	42.7
VAT	6.0	22.0	14.0	15.0	7.0	8.0	5.0	0.0	0.9

Note: B = Belgium; DK = Denmark; FRG = West Germany; F = France; I = Italy; NL = Netherlands; P = Portugal; E = Spain.

INDIRECT AND DIRECT MARKET INTERVENTIONS

Real, assumed and alleged special features of the pharmaceutical market (third party payment, price elasticity, transparency, oligopolistic structure, physicians' behaviour, etc.) and the fact that health is looked upon as a special good has led to increased public intervention in the health sector and especially in the pharmaceutical market. The increase of health care costs and their rising share of Gross National Product have led on occasion to the passing of political measures which were not always based on sound pricing considerations.

There are several different approaches which influence the

allocation of money for drug therapy and therefore the composition of health care services. One approach is to counter the alleged monopolies of the pharmaceutical companies by some countervailing power, i.e. create state or para-state monopsonies. However, if the state is too stringent as a monopsonist, capital will no longer be invested in this industry. According to economic theory, 'the outcome of the price determination process is indeterminate and rests on the relative power of the two sides' (Maynard, 1975). The situation in the United Kingdom tends towards this, although to date with a reasonable monopsist.

There are three different approaches to interventions which are used either separately or in combination: regulation of the overall consumption; direct or indirect quality restrictions; direct or indirect price interventions. The *total consumption* is controlled in Germany (for example) where any increase in drug consumption is collectively agreed upon at the beginning of the year. If the total consumption is higher than this agreed ceiling, physicians are individually advised whether they have overprescribed in terms of quantities or drugs which are too expensive. With this budget approach, the quantities of drugs as well as their prices are indirectly controlled. This may induce the physician to prescribe the cheaper drugs of the non-research-based companies. However, as long as the physicians are free to prescribe what they want there is no direct intervention in the competitive process of innovative and imitative firms.

The *quantities* are indirectly controlled in those countries where the state defines, either in a positive way the drugs whose costs are refunded totally or partially by the Social Security System (positive lists) or in a negative way those drugs whose costs are not refunded (negative lists). Figure 17.9 shows what different types of list exist today. Positive and negative lists are 'market entry lists'. These have no direct impact on the competitive process between innovative and imitative companies. However, their pricing and health policy effect is dubious. Physicians may substitute products which are not eligible for cost refunds by products which are. If the non-refundable products are less 'severe' products (e.g. natural compounds) then an adequate minor therapy is substituted by an unnecessarily major therapy. Normally the major therapy is more expensive than the minor one. These lists may therefore lead to medically inadequate and even more expensive drug therapies, although they were introduced to reduce costs to Social Security.[1]

Another means of influencing the amount of drug consumption is through the introduction of prescription fees for the consumer. This

Figure 17.9: Types of drug lists

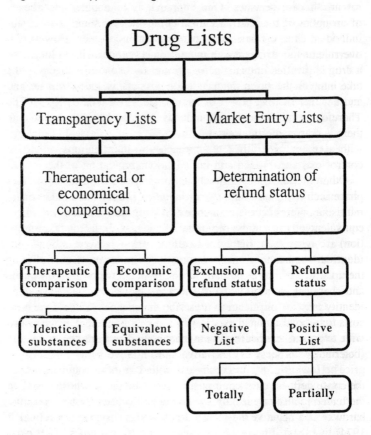

mechanism works only for a short time, either because consumers become accustomed to it or because inflation reduces the real amount of this fee over time. A possibility for further discussions should be the introduction of a 'health prime rate mechanism'. Government should increase the amount of cost sharing for the consumer if health care expenses grow too fast, and reduce if if they fall below the predicted rate. This tool would not distort the relative prices of health care products and services (because the private share of health care expenses would have to be paid for in any kind of health service) and could be flexibly adjusted like the prime rate in the monetary system.

The market entry lists, in addition to their extended quantitative effect, also have a direct effect on *prices*. If a preparation of a research-based company is only 'listed' if its price meets the price of an imitator, this restrains the competitive process, because the individual decision processes of physicians in the market place are overruled by an expert committee which decides whether a price for a drug is justified or not. Such an evaluation can, necessarily, only take into consideration the hardware of a drug (the physical entity) and not the software (i.e. the services rendered with the product). Therefore, even if the market were ready to pay for these services, there is no possibility of entering the market of refundable products with a price higher than the generic prices. (This sort of price control exists in France and the Netherlands.)

Other means of dealing with the assumed inefficiencies of the pharmaceutical market are the *transparency lists* where either only multisource products (i.e. identical substances) or therapeutically equivalent products (i.e. different substances for the same indication) are compared. There are several pitfalls with both lists. Even identical substances may have differences in quality and therapeutical effect in human bodies. The assumption of physical and chemical identity does not necessarily mean that an economic identity exists. Confidence in a product saves individual information costs for a physician and may justify a higher price. Therefore, even with identical hardware (homogeneous substances) the software (heterogeneous services) may differ and thus justify differences in prices. However, the justification is normally done individually by the consumer — expert committees have a tendency to compare (by the '*ceteris paribus* rule') only the hardware and select the cheapest hardware on offer as the most economic therapy (see Hoppmann, 1974).

Even more questionable from an economic point of view are price comparisons of heterogeneous but more or less therapeutically equivalent drugs. By their very nature they lead to price comparisons of heterogeneous products, comparisons which are inadequate from the economic point of view if one does not take account of all the relevant physical and service criteria of a product. Needless to say each consumer's weight will differ. These lists may help to increase the therapeutic and economic transparency for the physician as long as they are used voluntarily. They may reduce competition when they become the basis for compulsory substitution.

PROSPECTS AND CONCLUSIONS

Health care expenditures in the past have risen over-proportionally to the Gross National Product. This is a well-known fact. Estimates for the future do not predict an essential change of this past experience. For 1992 it is predicted that the share of public finance health care expenditure in the US will rise to 12.5 per cent of the GNP. The corresponding figure for France is 9.5 per cent, for Japan 9.0 per cent, for Germany 8.9 per cent. Parallel to that, worldwide growth of national economies is expected to rise by 21 per cent between 1982 and 1992 (see Figure 17.10). Obviously — as already stated at the beginning — the question of the allocation of resources and the pricing of medicines will gain even more importance.

Having discussed the fact that certain peculiarities of the pharmaceutical market may result in some inherent inefficiencies, it is clear that some other forms of market interference with respect to pharmaceutical prices can be expected in the future. The actual forms of price controls for pharmaceuticals is demonstrated in a simplified way in Figure 17.11.

Figure 17.10: Health care expenditures and economic growth

HCE in % of GNP/GDP

	1982	1992
US	10.5	12.5
France	8.4	9.6
Japan	5.1	9.0
Germany	8.5	8.9
Italy	6.3	7.4
Spain	6.2	6.8
UK	6.3	6.4

Average annual real GNP growth 1882-92 in %

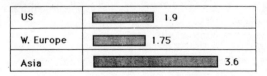

US	1.9
W. Europe	1.75
Asia	3.6

Figure 17.11: Price control in the EEC

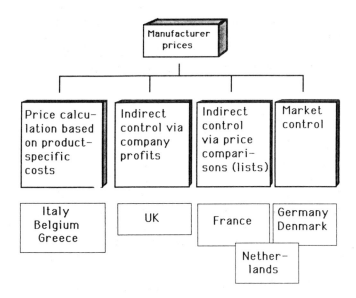

The competitive process between research-based and non-research-based companies achieved a balance as long as the research-based companies had a constant flow of new products. Their temporary competitive advantage of obtaining higher prices and profits was threatened by other research-based companies and non-research-based companies. Both competitive processes controlled prices and profits.

Public intervention to control pharmaceutical costs began at a time when the research-based industry had reached a more complex stage. The form of state intervention did not correct the inefficiencies of the market but sometimes created even more inefficiencies.

Lessons that could be drawn from experiences gained so far for all participants in the health care system can be summarised as follows:

1. Countries start with different levels of supply, structures and socio-political environments. It would be fallacious just to 'copy' a regulatory approach in one country without taking into regard all relevant components.

2. Incremental approaches in the various health care sectors have

247

dominated over the synoptic approach. Thus none of the countries with an established social security system has achieved more than alleviation of the symptoms of cost explosion.

3. Most countries have selected the prices of medicines as the politically easiest target of intervention, though it was by no means the most important one in terms of potential savings.

4. Nearly all types of health care regulation are based on control measures. Incentive approaches, i.e. a voluntary economic use of health resources by the supply and demand side have hitherto been neglected; e.g. Health Maintenance Organisations, competitive insurance plans, new forms of cost-sharing, etc.

5. Cost containment measures ensuring the future financing of the health care sector are legitimate and necessary. All parties engaged in the health care sector (i.e. physicians, patients and the pharmaceutical industry) will have to contribute to achieve this objective.

6. A system of safeguarding an innovative climate in a competitive environment would therefore be in the best interest of both consumer and industry.

NOTE

1. For a good survey of cost containment in the EEC countries see: Abel-Smith, B. and Grandjeat, P. (1978) 'Pharmaceutical consumption: trends in expenditure: main measures taken and underlying objectives of public intervention in this field'. *Social Policy Series, no. 38*, Office for Official Publications of the European Community, Luxembourg, Brussels, p. 58.

REFERENCES

Bureau of Consumer Protection (1979) *Drug product selection*. Staff Report to the Federal Trade Commission, Washington, p. 14.
Chamberlin, E.H. (1933) *The theory of monopolistic competition*. Cambridge.
Clark, J.M. (1940) 'Towards a concept of workable competition'. *American Economic Review, 30*, p. 241.
——— (1961) *Competition as a dynamic process*. The Brooking Institution, Washington, pp. 180–1.
Feldstein, P.J. (1979) *Health care economics*. Wiley Medical, New York, pp. 4–10.

Hoppmann, E. (1974) *Die Abgrenzung des relevanten Marktes im Rahmen der Missbrauchsaufsicht über marktbeherrschende Unternehmen dargestellt am Beispiel der Praxis des Bundeskartellamtes bei Arzneimitteln.* Nomos Verlagsgesellschaft, Baden-Baden, p. 122.

Langle, L. *et al.* (1985) 'Le cout d'un nouveau médicament'. *Journal d'Economie médical*, 2, 1.

Lipsey, R.G. and Steiner, P.O. (1978) *Economics*, 5th edn. Harper and Row, New York, p. 15.

Maynard, A. (1975) *Health care in the European community.* Croom Helm, London, p. 269.

Penrose, E.T. (1968) *The theory of the growth of a firm.* Blackwell and Mott, Oxford, p. 264.

Reekie, D.W. (1977) *Pricing new pharmaceutical products.* Macmillan, London.

―――― (1978) 'Price and quality competition in the United States drug industry'. *J. Ind. Econ.*, 26, 223.

Rosenberg, L.J. (1977) *Marketing.* Prentice-Hall, Englewood Cliffs, NJ, p. 350.

Simon, H. (1982) 'Preispolitik im Pharmamarkt'. *Pharma-Marketing-journal*, 4, 140.

Slatter, St.O. (1977) *Competition and marketing strategies in the pharmaceutical industry.* Croom Helm, London, p. 18.

Stahl, I. (1979) *Health care and drug development. Production and productivity developments in the health sector.* University of Lund, Sweden.

Weston, J.F. (1979) 'Pricing in the pharmaceutical industry'. In R.I. Chien (ed.), *Issues in pharmaceutical economics.* Lexington Books, Lexington, Mass., p. 76.

18

Pharmaceutical Competition

Thi Dao

EVOLUTION IN PHARMACEUTICAL COMPETITION

Competition in the pharmaceutical industry is a multi-dimensional concept. While some economists speak of different elements of competition, such as price competition, product competition, promotional competition and generic competition (Reekie, 1975; Kahn *et al.*, 1982), critics of the industry maintain that competition should be used to refer only to price competition; whereas the other elements of competition are called 'rivalry' (Schifrin, 1982). This latter sentiment, of course, reflects a deep allegiance to an economic theory in which competition is defined in terms of prices and outputs that relate to static efficiency — a situation without growth or technological progress. The pharmaceutical industry, however, is research-intensive and operates on the basis of growth via innovation. Therefore, it is clearly not appropriate to define competition on the same basis as static efficiency. In fact, according to the Schumpeterian hypothesis, it is quite possible that price competition may be inversely related to progressiveness. And this is because consumer welfare, which is affected by innovation, may not be served by the maximum degree of price competition (Comanor, 1979).

For the purposes of this chapter, competition is given a broader meaning than just price competition. In fact, price competition and product competition are viewed as the two extremes of the spectrum, while the other elements of competition are treated as secondary issues dominated by them. For example, promotional competition is essentially driven by product competition, its focus being to differentiate one product from another. Generic competition, on the other hand, is simply price competition between an original product and its generic versions. Schematically, pharmaceutical competition can be presented as follows:

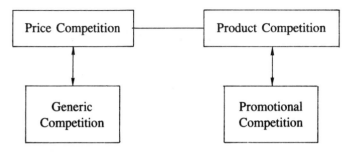

Until recently, pharmaceutical competition focused mostly on product differentiation. Companies maintained their market positions by producing new drugs whose therapeutic value could be distinguished from those already in existence. New drugs, therefore, have been the lifeblood of the industry. In the context of health care systems where physicians alone dictated the delivery of health care without much concern about its costs, product competition was consistent with the needs of physicians and patients alike. Physicians wanted to have a wide range of choices of therapies, whereas patients were able to try almost anything that was available and perhaps more suitable to their specific conditions.

This situation, however, began to change in all industrialised countries in the mid-1970s. As the growth in health care expenditures continued to outpace the growth of the economy, cost-containment policies were implemented in most countries to make more efficient use of available economic resources. As some observers of the industry have remarked, cost containment pressures have put an end to the idea that health care should be provided by an individual doctor to an individual patient according to the 'freedom of the doctor to choose the best medicine for his patient' principle (*Scrip*, 25 December, 1985). The need to achieve the best value for money, i.e. cost-effectiveness, has forced a change in the focus of health care from serving the needs of the individual to serving the population as a whole. The idiosyncratic differences among patients are played down and the focus is on problems associated with the 'average' patient. With this development, the role of physicians in the delivery of health care has begun to change. They are no longer the only decision makers. Their influence on the choice of pharmaceuticals is increasingly being compromised by clinical

251

pharmacologists, pharmacists, programme administrators, financial managers and even patients themselves. Because the interest of these decision makers is mainly to be cost-effective, pharmaceutical competition based exclusively on product differentiation has ceased to be effective.

As would be expected, however, pharmaceutical companies did not immediately go from product competition to price competition. Instead, to meet the cost-containment needs of decision makers, traditional information on a medicine's safety and efficacy is now often accompanied by cost-effectiveness data. (See Appendix for a brief discussion of what cost-effectiveness means and how it is related to the characteristics of a medicine.) By the end of 1985, advertisements in professional journals in the US clearly demonstrated companies' interest in using cost-effectiveness to differentiate their products. A good example is this advertisement in many issues of the *New England Journal of Medicine* concerning Rocephin by Hoffman-LaRoche: '*Cost-effective* . . . substantial savings provided by once-a-day dosage and reduced administration costs — outpatient management offers an additional opportunity for cost containment'. In the United Kingdom, highlighting the quality-of-life effects of medicines appears to be the preferred approach. For example, both Squibb and Merck & Co. featured the quality-of-life issue in promotional material for their respective anti-hypertensive compounds, captopril and enalapril (*Scrip*, 1 July, 1985).

With the use of cost-effectiveness data, a linkage has been created between product competition and price competition. Because the basis for demonstrating the cost effectiveness of a medicine often involves superior efficacy and/or superior safety which bring about significant savings in terms of costs associated with hospitalisation and medical/surgical procedures, a cost-effective medicine could justify a higher price than its competitor(s). The lack of cost-effectiveness evidence, on the other hand, would mean that the medicine does not offer therapeutic and/or safety advantage over its competitor(s). In this case, it is likely that reimbursement authorities (or the market) will force the medicine's marketer to accept a low price.

Other concurrent developments have also helped push pharmaceutical companies further in the direction of price competition. Most important among them is the increasing use of generics in many countries. In 1984 the US Congress passed the Drug Price Competition and Patent Term Restoration Act. Because this legislation is designed partly to foster generic competition, it is widely perceived as a door-opener for many generic companies to enter the US market which, thus far, has been dominated by the research-intensive companies. In the UK, the advent of limited lists of reimbursable medicines in 1985 has provided a significant push for increasing use of generics in some therapeutic areas. In West Germany, increasing pressure is found in the form of withholding payment from physicians who prescribe the original brand instead of a generic.

PHARMACEUTICAL COMPETITION IN THE FUTURE

During the coming decades, pharmaceutical competition will be intense. Whether a company chooses to participate in the innovative product markets or in the generic markets, or both, it will be faced with intense competition. Further, the nature of the competition in each of these market segments will be very different from that of today. As cost-containment pressures continue to push for lower prices, fundamental changes will take place in the way companies carry out their research and development (R&D) efforts and market their products. Moreover, some research-intensive companies will also feel the pressure to expand their traditional mission and to reduce the impact of generic competition by participating in the generic market themselves.

Despite all these changes, however, it is important to remember that innovative products hold the key to a research-intensive pharmaceutical company's future and its profitability. For, unlike generics, new products can offer new therapeutic value for which society is unwilling to pay high prices. More importantly, these prices are protected because as new medicines continue to be protected by patents in the industrialised world, the originators will be able to prevent any price competition from generics for the duration of the patent terms.

Product competition based on cost-effectiveness

The stakes in product competition will significantly increase. As decision makers increasingly seek economic efficiency, traditional sources of revenue for pharmaceutical companies will dry up. First, as a result of the US Drug Price Competition and Patent Term Restoration Act of 1984, it is expected that a medicine — especially

253

one with significant market success — will be faced with generic competition as soon as its patent expires. Any revenue that in the past might have been realised due to a delay in generic competition, therefore, would be lost. Secondly, originator companies are likely to suffer revenue loss whether they decide to cut prices and remain competitive to generics or maintain prices and lose a greater proportion of market share.

To compete effectively in the future marketplace, however, pharmaceutical companies need more than just new medicines — they need new medicines that are cost-effective. Product competition based on cost-effectiveness will have a significant impact on the way companies do business and their collective and individual public image. At the industry level, the cost-effectiveness standard will preempt any need for governments to institute new price controls. For, as a mechanism by which medicines can be differentiated (by therapeutic benefits and/or quantified economic values), cost-effectiveness is, in effect, a form of economic regulation.

And with this mechanism, product competition can take only one of the two following forms: first, if a new medicine is found to be more cost-effective than its competitors, the marketer can justify a higher price. Further, the medicine is likely to enjoy a leading market position because its cost-effectiveness will induce decision makers to grant it 'medicine-of-choice' status. Second, if the therapeutic and safety benefits offered by the medicine are not sufficient to make it more cost-effective than existing competitors, its marketer will be forced to accept a lower price.

From a societal viewpoint, this development should be viewed as very positive. When pharmaceutical companies decide that it is in their interest to engage in product competition based on the cost-effectiveness concept, they have adopted, in effect, a form of economic regulation without the cumbersome administration and high costs often associated with government controls. Scarce economic resources, therefore, could be saved or used more efficiently. This contribution to economic efficiency will not be limited to the US, where most of companies' cost-effectiveness studies have been undertaken. Because of the multinational nature of the pharmaceutical industry and the similar nature of cost-containment concerns around the world, it is reasonable to expect that the cost-effectiveness standard will also be accepted outside the US — most likely the industrialised world — in the foreseeable future.

From the perspective of a pharmaceutical company, product competition based on cost-effectiveness will significantly change the way it markets products and, perhaps to a lesser extent, the way it conducts R&D. To satisfy the cost-effectiveness standard in the marketplace, companies will need to incorporate cost-effectiveness studies early in the process of a new medicine's development. Although research staff currently tend to resist the use of economic criteria as a basis for R&D funding, companies will be increasingly sensitive to the market potential of an R&D project. While it is not clear to what extent the cost-effectiveness potential of a medicine will become the overriding basis for an R&D project either to be carried to fruition or terminated in its early phases, it is reasonable to believe that R&D activities in the future will be influenced by market environments where hard scientific and economic data constitute the basis for success.

Generic competition

As a result of many developments, perhaps the most important of which is the US Drug Price Competition and Patent Term Restoration Act of 1984, observers of the pharmaceutical industry are unanimous about the potential growth of generics in the future. In the US, a study recently estimated that annual sales of generics will reach US$ 8.5 million by 1990, giving generics a 35 per cent share of the market (Schaumann, 1985). In this same year, another US researcher estimated that 80 per cent of the top 200 prescription drugs will face generic competition (Grabowski, quoted in *IMS Pharmaceutical Newsletter*, 15 July, 1985). As pointed out earlier, generic competition is essentially price competition between pioneer products and their generic versions. Intensified generic competition, therefore, means that revenue generated by medicines whose patents have expired will be significantly reduced. Unless a pioneer company can produce new medicines in time to serve as alternative sources of income, generic competition can be devastating to the company in the short run. A good example was the widely publicised situation encountered by Hoffmann-LaRoche when Valium's patent expired in 1985 (*Economist*, 23 February, 1985).

To deal with generic competition, some research-intensive companies have created generic subsidiaries to minimise the potential loss of revenue to their generic competitors. In the US, A.H. Robins, Ciba-Geigy, and Boehringer — to name just a few — have either acquired or established their generic companies. Other major companies have long adopted the approach of using their own names

255

in lines of branded generics; for example, Smith Kline's SK-Line, Lederle's Standard Products and Parke Davis' generic line. Further penetration of the generic market by pioneer companies is expected in the future as these companies struggle to recover eroding sales.

Despite pioneer companies' participation in the generic market, however, many have predicted that the structure of the industry in the future will be two-tiered, with the innovative products being in the top tier and the generic business the secondary segment. This is because profits in the generic business are likely to be very small compared to those that significant breakthroughs can generate.

From a marketing viewpoint, generic competition and product competition based on cost-effectiveness have at least one thing in common. That is, when a new medicine turns out to be less cost-effective than its competitor(s), competition will be in terms of price despite patent protection.

CONCLUSION

Because of developments in the marketplace, pharmaceutical competition in the future will be markedly different to that of today. As opposed to the current dichotomy where generic competition focuses exclusively on prices and therapeutic competition on product differentiation, one will see price competition even among therapeutic alternatives. The pharmaceutical industry's adoption of the cost-effectiveness standard will make it the driving force behind competition. If a new medicine can be demonstrated to be more cost-effective than its therapeutic alternative(s), it can be a 'big winner' because it can justify a high price and a leading market position. Otherwise, it will be a 'big loser', and could only survive on the market if it is price competitive. In this regard, the new medicine will not be different from a generic product.

Schematically, pharmaceutical competition in the future can be presented as follows:

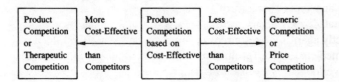

Product Competition or Therapeutic Competition	More Cost-Effective than Competitors	Product Competition based on Cost-Effective	Less Cost-Effective than Competitors	Generic Competition or Price Competition

From a public policy perspective, product competition based on cost-effectiveness should be viewed as a development with the potential to improve economic efficiency in health care without government intervention. Because of the innovative nature of the pharmaceutical development process and the high R&D costs associated with a new medicine, this market-based competition is far superior to any government policies which may be designed for the same purpose — for nothing except the 'invisible hand' of the market can approximate the balance between economic efficiency and innovation.

APPENDIX: COST-EFFECTIVENESS OF DRUG THERAPY

Generally speaking, cost-effectiveness means achieving a desired health outcome at the lowest possible cost. Implicit in the cost-effectiveness concept, therefore, is a comparison of one pharmaceutical therapy against another, or one pharmaceutical therapy against another mode of treatment, such as surgery. But what is the framework for such comparison?

Based on the economic concept of resource utilisation, the framework consists of not only medicines but the health care system and society at large. Strictly speaking, the cost-effectiveness of a medicine must be assessed by comparing total consumption against savings in pharmaceutical costs, health care resources, and productive capital (e.g. work productivity) that result from its use. This comparison must be done for each of the medicines involved in the assessment. The net consumption (or savings) associated with each medicine will, in turn, be compared; and the one with the lowest net consumption (or highest net savings) will be identified as the most cost-effective product. (For a detailed discussion on the cost-effectiveness methodology, see Dao, 1985.)

Another aspect of the cost-effectiveness concept in health care involves the effects of a pharmaceutical therapy on patients' quality of life. Improvements in quality of life resulting from alleviation of pain and more freedom of movement, however, cannot easily be evaluated in monetary terms. Therefore, they cannot be compared directly against the resource consumption necessitated by the use of the medicine. As a result, important benefits of the medicine may be overlooked by decision makers who are more preoccupied with cost containment. To correct this situation, efforts have been made to assess systematically the quality-of-life effects of pharmaceutical therapy and to call them to the attention of decision makers (Smith, 1983; Wenger, Mattson, Furberg and Elinson, 1984). Quality of life as used in this context refers broadly to patients' physical, mental and psychological abilities to maintain their usual daily activities.

Because cost-effectiveness is nothing more than a translation of a product's characteristics into an aggregate economic value, product characteristics form the basis for cost-effectiveness demonstration. A cost-effective product must have superiority in at least one of the following areas — provided that everything else is basically similar to its competitor: efficacy; safety; dosing frequency; price.

It should be pointed out that when price is used as the main thrust of the cost-effectiveness argument, everything else being the same, it is almost impossible for competitors to come up with a cost-effectiveness counterposition. The most vivid example of this situation is competition between generics and brand name medicines. Unless it can be demonstrated that generics are poorer in quality — and therefore inferior in safety and efficacy — their generally lower prices mean that price competition is inevitable.

REFERENCES

Comanor, W. (1979) 'Competition in the pharmaceutical industry'. In R.I. Chien (ed.), *Issues in pharmaceutical economics*. D.C. Heath, Lexington, Mass.

Dao, T.D. (1985) 'Cost-benefit and cost-effectiveness analysis of drug therapy'. *American Journal of Hospital Pharmacy*, 42, 4, 791–802.

Kahn, P., Young, E.J., Egan, J.W., *et al.* (1982) *Economics of the pharmaceutical industry*. Praeger, New York.

Reekie, D. (1975) *The economics of the pharmaceutical industry*. Macmillan, London.

Schaumann, L. (1985) *Pharmaceutical industry perspectives: a generics milestone* (vol. 1). SRI International, Menlo Park.

Schifrin, L. (1982) Comments made at the Project HOPE workshop on *The effectiveness of medicines in containing health care costs: impact of innovation, regulation and quality*, edited by the National Pharmaceutical Council, Washington, D.C.

Smith, G.T. (ed.) (1983) *Measuring the social benefits of medicine*. Office of Health Economics, London.

Wenger, N.K., Mattson, M.E., Furberg, C.D. and Elinson, J. (eds) (1984) *Assessment of quality of life in clinical trials of cardiovascular therapies*. Le Jacq, New York.

19

Pharmaceutical Regulation: The Past and Future Twenty-five Years

Ronald Hansen

INTRODUCTION

The 25th anniversary of the founding of the Office of Health Economics in the United Kingdom coincides with the 25th anniversary of legislation which significantly altered the process of regulating pharmaceutical innovations in the United States. The years since the passage of the 1962 Amendments to the Food Drug and Cosmetics Act have witnessed major changes in the pharmaceutical industry and in the worldwide regulations which affect it. This joint anniversary is an appropriate time to reflect on the past and future of pharmaceutical regulation and its implications for the industry.

This essay will focus on regulatory developments in the United States primarily because these are the most familiar to the author. It should be noted that while the specifics of the regulations and the timing of their introduction differ among countries, viewed in a broad perspective, there are many similarities in the regulatory trends in western countries. Moreover, since the large innovative firms are multinational and look to the international market-place in their development decisions, changes in regulations affecting major markets will affect the innovative activities in other markets even if their regulations remain unchanged.

The regulation of pharmaceutical products in the United States began early in the century, well before the development of the modern industry. In the US, the 1906 Pure Food and Drugs Act, passed during the era of patent medicines, was designed to ensure proper labelling of any substance used to treat disease. The Sherley Amendment in 1912 prohibited fraudulent claims, but this provision was weakened by a Supreme Court ruling that if the manufacturer believed his product was effective for all claimed uses, then the claims could not be considered fraudulent.

The deaths of approximately 100 people who used Elixir Sulfanilamide containing a lethal solvent resulted in the passage of the Food, Drug and Cosmetics Act of 1938. This not only further restricted labelling and advertising but also introduced the requirement that new drugs be approved as safe by the Food and Drug Administration (FDA) before being marketed. The modern pharmaceutical industry, which can be considered to have been in its infancy at this time, has been subject to premarketing approval regulations in the US for most of its existence. Similar requirements did not appear in Great Britain until substantially later. For a more extensive history of early US legislation, the reader should consult Peter Temin's *Taking Your Medicine* (1980).

The thalidomide tragedy dramatically raised public concern about the possible adverse effects of pharmaceuticals. Even if the episode had not resulted in any formal legislative changes, it would have undoubtedly changed the manner in which pharmaceutical firms, regulators and the public viewed new drugs and the pharmaceutical development process. In Great Britain, the Minister of Health established the Safety of Drugs Committee. Although the arrangement was initially voluntary, the Proprietary Association of Great Britain and the Association of the British Pharmaceutical Industry promised that none of their members would conduct clinical trials or market new drugs without the Committee's approval (Dunlop, 1973). In the United States the tragedy is credited with providing the spark that resulted in a major overhaul of US drug regulations, even though some critics have claimed that the 1962 Amendments probably would have done little to prevent the episode had they been in effect.

One of the principal additions to the regulations incorporated in the 1962 Amendments was the requirement that a drug must be shown to be efficacious as well as safe. Moreover, claims which firms make about their drugs must receive approval from the FDA. Showing efficacy often requires large-scale and lengthy studies particularly in some therapeutic areas.

Another important aspect of the 1962 Amendments was the requirement that firms receive an investigational new drug exemption (IND) from the FDA prior to the initiation of clinical trials. This meant not only that firms had to apply formally to the FDA, but also that the FDA became involved with all drugs clinically examined and not just those eventually submitted for approval. Moreover, this involvement started prior to clinical trials rather than at the end.

260

Essentially, the FDA became involved in the process of testing as well as in the review of the testing results.

While the 1962 Amendments marked a major milestone in US drug regulations, the actual change was not as abrupt as it is sometimes said to have been. It required considerable time for the FDA to implement changes and for the firms to adjust to them. In fact, there has been a process of almost continuous change since 1962 even though the underlying statuatory authority has remained virtually unchanged.

Several major changes in the performance of the pharmaceutical industry coincide with the regulatory change although other influences have affected some of the observed trends. The number of new drugs tested on man in the US declined steadily during the early part of the period. The trend shows signs of levelling off but at a much lower point than previously. New drug approvals, which averaged around 40 per year prior to 1962, dropped to an average close to 15 per year. Whether 1985's record 23 approvals is a sign of a reversal of this trend, or just a temporary blip, remains to be seen. The length of time required from first human testing to marketing approval had steadily increased to eight years by 1979 (Wardell, May and Trimble, 1982) and some estimates place the figure at 10 years for drugs approved recently. As a result of the lengthy testing process, the time remaining on the original patent at the point of marketing approval, usually referred to as the effective patent life, has steadily declined to less than 10 years (Eisman and Wardell, 1981). The cost of drug development has also risen significantly, from somewhere under $10 million prior to 1962, to $54 million for drugs first tested in man between 1963 and 1975 (Hansen, 1979). Estimates place the average near $100 million today though no rigorous study has been made recently.

FUTURE TRENDS

It is always difficult to make predictions about the specific course of pharmaceutical regulation, in part, because past changes have been affected by episodes such as the sulfamide poisonings and the thalidomide tragedy which would be difficult to predict. Also, the regulatory climate is affected by political events which are difficult enough for political scientists to predict. Nevertheless, we will attempt to project from current conditions to future events.

With conservative governments in the US, UK, and Canada and

261

some signs of a retrenchment from socialist policies in much of continental Europe, one would be tempted to predict an easing of drug regulations. Deregulation has been a major issue in the US for over a decade and even made advances during the Carter administration. Similar trends have emerged in much of Europe. Should we be so bold as to predict a deregulation of drug development? And if drug development is deregulated, will the trends noted above be reserved?

If one looks carefully at the deregulation that has taken place in the US, what one observes is not general deregulation, but a shift in the nature of regulation. One could group industrial regulations into two broad categories: price and quantity regulations and health and safety regulations. Almost all of the deregulation falls into the former category. For example, entry and pricing restrictions in the telecommunications, trucking and airline industries have been reduced. The regulations governing the financial services industry have been substantially changed. Although price and entry restrictions have been declining, health and safety regulations have been increasing. Despite charges that the current administration has been lax in its enforcement duties, during the past two decades a wide range of environmental protection, occupational safety and health regulations have been introduced. Deregulation may more properly be reregulation and the recent trends do not point to any significant reduction in the stringency of drug regulations.

Examining recent legislative and regulatory changes affecting the pharmaceutical industry, one observes changes that have affected financial and administrative conditions, but not the fundamental safety and efficacy issues. The lengthening development times and increased cost of development raised concerns about the viability of pharmaceutical innovation but the remedies which have been implemented have not significantly affected drug regulation. In order to encourage the development of drugs intended for rare conditions, with little market potential despite their importance to a small number of patients, Congress passed the Orphan Drug Act. This bill gives tax credits to firms who pursue the development of these drugs. The decline in effective patent protection caused by longer development times was offset by the Drug Price Competition and Patent Term Restoration Act which granted some restoration of patent protection based on the length of time the drug was in the regulatory process and the time which otherwise remained on the patent. As part of the same act the only significant deregulatory initiative was established but this affected generic drugs not new innovations. The act clarified the requirements for approval of generic versions of previously approved drugs and thus reduced the testing requirements relative to past FDA practice. Except for this last provision, Congressional action has focussed on addressing the financial aspects of stricter regulations rather than on deregulating the drug approval process.

The Food and Drug Administration has engaged in several actions designed to affect the performance of the drug approval process. The changes, many of which have fallen short of their initial promise, focus on administrative procedures rather than on reduced testing requirements or changes in risk assessment parameters. The FDA has been willing to give more weight to foreign clinical trials, has initiated a fast-track system for new drugs it considers important (presumably a slow track for others though that it not explicit) and has rewritten the regulations governing the review process for new drug applications (NDAs). Opinions differ on whether these changes have had or are likely to have a significant effect on the time required for new drug testing.

Are we likely to observe any significant changes in the new drug approval process in the future? While there will certainly be a variety of administrative changes, I do not anticipate any relaxation of drug approval requirements so long as the basic structure of the FDA and public perceptions and attitudes about risk remain unchanged. Asymmetries in the information available about potential new therapies generate incentives which slow the approval process. Approved drugs which are later linked to adverse effects will often create public and Congressional complaints about poor performance at the FDA. New therapies which are still in the regulatory pipeline are largely unknown to the public, Congress or even many members of the medical community. Failure to speedily approve these drugs rarely generates criticism of FDA performance even though some potential beneficiaries are denied access to improved therapies. Given these incentives, one should not be surprised that individuals at the FDA are likely to be very cautious about new drug approvals. We should rather be thankful that the system generates as many approvals as it does.

Public attitudes about risk and the responsibility for assuming risk is revealed through another channel which also significantly affects pharmaceutical products. While not directly a form of drug regulation, product liability statutes impose some of the same constraints on drug firms as direct regulation. Firms which market unsafe, ineffective or fraudulently advertised products are subject to liability for damages which these actions generate. To avoid liability claims, firms must review the performance of their products in much the same way as required by regulatory authorities. The major differences are that firms would be free to select their own testing and evaluation methods and, unless specifically prohibited by the courts, product liability does not prohibit the marketing of unsafe or ineffective drugs, although it does make it expensive to the firm to do so. Thus product liability imposes decisions on the firms about marketing which are similar to the criteria used for regulatory approval. Depending on their relative stringency, liability rules may obviate the effects of regulation or vice versa. Thus, we would be remiss to consider the effects of one without considering the effects of the other. Moreover, changes in product liability statutes may portend changes in regulations since many of the same forces which operate to shape liability statutes also establish the regulatory rules.

United States product liability laws have shown changes which parallel the changes in drug regulations. Prior to the late 1950s, a victim of a defective product had to establish not only that the product was defective but also that the defendant was negligent. In fact, in many instances, it was not possible to sue the manufacturer directly since the consumer's contractual arrangement was viewed to be with the retailer. Since that time several developments in US product liability rules have increased the liability exposure of manufacturers, including drug manufacturers. One may now directly sue the manufacturer, class action suits have proliferated, and increasingly decisions are based on strict liability rather than negligence. When bodily injury is involved, the awards for pain and suffering or punitive damages often exceed the estimates of direct economic harm. At the present time, there is considerable talk of a liability crisis with charges and counter-charges about whether increases in liability insurance rates are due to the increase in expected liability exposure or due to price gouging by the insurance industry. Whatever the truth of that debate, many activities are being restricted due to concerns about liability exposure.

Pharmaceutical firms have not been immune from product liability problems. In some instances, they were protected by provisions of the statutes which specifically reduced liability for new pharmaceuticals which were considered inherently hazardous but socially beneficial. The manufacturer, despite rigorous testing, could not reasonably be expected to be aware of all hazards since some would become apparent only with extensive use or the passage of time. The case law is changing in this dimension as well, with court decisions moving closer to strict liability.

Product liability concerns are clearly playing an important role in drug development and marketing. One of the areas which has recently been of great concern, is the use of vaccines (Kirch, 1985). Even though many vaccines have been approved by the FDA, and in many cases marketed for substantial periods of time, their continued production and use is threatened by product liability problems. Lederle Laboratories was unable to obtain insurance coverage for its DTP vaccine after several lawsuits alleging that the vaccine was responsible for brain damage to infants resulted in large awards to the plaintiffs. The company has recently announced that it will continue to market the vaccine, but will substantially increase the price in order to offset its liability exposure. Many other firms have stopped producing vaccines entirely and there is concern that some vaccines may simply become unavailable. Another product which has been the target of several lawsuits is Benedictin, a drug which is used to relieve morning sickness. Although the drug has FDA approval and has been marketed for many years, its manufacturer, Merrell Dow, has removed the drug from the market, citing its liability exposure as the primary reason. Product liability statutes are similar to a second layer of regulation and have significantly curtailed pharmaceutical innovation in areas considered to be vulnerable to high liability exposure.

The current characterisation of the product liability situation as a 'crisis' offers the prospect of legislative changes which may significantly alter the situation. California recently reduced the amount which could be awarded for pain and suffering and other states have legislation pending which will alter their liability statutes. If these changes result in a major reduction in the liability exposure for pharmaceutical firms then the effects of this secondary form of regulation will be reduced. Of potentially greater importance is the possibility that the current discussion of liability and risk-taking may generate a change in the public perception of how risks should be shared. If it generates an attitude that some activities are inherently risky but are nevertheless worthwhile and that government cannot, or possibly should not, try to protect individuals from all risks, then we may observe a change in the willingness to accept the potential risks of new drugs in order to obtain more or speedier new drug approvals. While this is certainly very speculative, the current discussion surrounding the 'liability crisis' offers a rare opportunity for a reversal of a trend in the United States towards reduced personal responsibility for risk-taking in health-related matters.

265

Whether or not fundamental changes occur in the structure of the drug approval process, drug regulation will be affected by the nature of the pharmaceuticals being developed. The products of genetic engineering and the new biotechnology industry are likely to require changes in regulatory oversight. For many of these products the process of synthesising and manufacturing is significantly different from that of more traditional pharmaceutical preparations. Regulatory authorities will have to establish new guidelines reflecting these differences. For example, questions about the stability of the complex chemical chains may require different types of testing procedures. Although chemical manufacturing has environmental implications, some of the substances being engineered, particularly those which are capable of reproduction, have raised new concerns about the potential for environmental damage. These concerns may require new restrictions not only on the manufacture of drugs but also on the distribution system and the administration of the drugs.

One area which is likely to receive more attention in the future is post-marketing surveillance. Since some effects of drugs are not apparent until after prolonged use, post-marketing studies are useful in detecting effects which may not appear in clinical trials. In some cases, the manner in which drugs are used in general practice differs from the administration in controlled clinical trials which also results in unexpected effects. Several critics argue that the US regulatory system does not adequately monitor drugs once they are approved.

Some individuals advocate an increase in post-marketing surveillance in return for a reduction in pre-marketing testing requirements. By adding a fourth phase to the testing process, the drug candidate could complete the first three pre-marketing phases faster and thus be available for marketing earlier. Some critics of this proposal fear that Phase 4 will simply be an add-on requirement and will not lessen pre-marketing requirements. Others worry that the implementation of Phase 4 may make consumers wary of utilising the drug; however, some proponents view this as a good result. It is likely that some increase in post-marketing surveillance will occur in the US. The effect on drug development and utilisation will depend on the form this programme takes.

Recent incidents of product tampering in the United States have raised a different level of concern about the safety of medications. While one could hope that this is a temporary problem, its potential recurrence has raised fears about the security of the manufacturing and distribution system. Whether changes in packaging and reductions in the use of capsules will alleviate the problem is currently an open question. If they do not, one should expect a greater role for regulators in overseeing the distribution system.

Greater international co-operation among drug regulatory agencies has often been suggested. The increased willingness to accept foreign clinical data does suggest the possibility of greater interaction among regulatory agencies. While there are economies to be realised by greater co-ordination, there are also serious costs involved. The current fragmentation of regulatory authorities results in a diversity of decisions and offers the potential of judging the performance of one regulatory system against another. If only a single decision making authority were responsible for the drug approval process, one would lose this ability to compare the performance of the regulator. Moreover, judging by the example of other large organisations, one should expect less flexibility and greater bureaucratic delays. Although I do anticipate greater regional co-ordination over the next few decades, I think that international co-operation will stop short of a single agency structure.

In summary, I expect that while there will be changes in the administrative structure of drug regulations, the underlying parameters are likely to remain similar. Barring a major change in the public's perception and attitude toward risk taking, there will not be a major deregulation of the drug approval process. A major drug-related catastrophe may even result in stricter standards. The major changes in drug regulations are likely to be produced by the new developments in genetic engineering. While greater co-operation among national regulatory authorities will occur, this effort will stop short of evolving into a single regulatory authority.

REFERENCES

Dunlop, Sir D. (1973) 'The British system of drug regulation'. In R.L. Landau (ed.), *Regulating new drugs*. University of Chicago, Center for Policy Study, Chicago, pp. 230–7.

Eisman, M.M. and Wardell, W.M. (1981) 'The decline in effective patent life of new drugs'. *Research Management*, 24, 1, 18–21.

Hansen, R.W. (1979) 'The pharmaceutical development process: estimates of development costs and times and the effects of proposed regulatory changes'. In R.I. Chien (ed.), *Issues in pharmaceutical economics*. D.C. Heath, Lexington, Mass.

Kirch, E.W. (1985) 'Vaccines and product liability: a case of contagious litigation'. *Regulation*, May/June, pp. 11–18.

Temin, P. (1980) *Taking your medicine: drug regulation in the United States*. Harvard University Press, Cambridge, Massachusetts and

London.

Wardell, W.M., May, M.S. and Trimble, A.G. (1982) 'New drug development by U.S. pharmaceutical firms with analyses of trends in the acquisition and origin of drug candidates, 1963–1979'. *Clinical Pharmacology and Therapeutics, 32*, 4, 407–17, St. Louis, Missouri.

Index